CONTEMPORARY ISSUES IN BIOETHICS

Edited by **Peter A. Clark**

Contemporary Issues in Bioethics
Edited by Peter A. Clark

Published by InTech
Janeza Trdine 9, 51000 Rijeka, Croatia

Publishing Process Manager Silvia Vlase

Technical Editor Teodora Smiljanic

Cover Designer InTech Design Team

Additional hard copies can be obtained from orders@intechopen.com

Contemporary Issues in Bioethics, Edited by Peter A. Clark
p. cm.
ISBN 978-953-51-0169-7

For EU product safety concerns:
IN TECH d.o.o., Prolaz Marije Krucifikse Kozulić 3, 51000 Rijeka, Croatia, info@intechopen.com or visit our website at intechopen.com.

Meet the editor

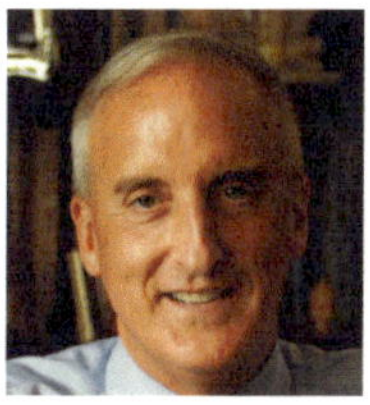

Peter A. Clark, S.J., Ph.D. is a Professor of Theology and Health Administration and Director of the Institute of Catholic Bioethics at Saint Joseph's University in Philadelphia, Pennsylvania. He is also the Bioethicist for the Mercy Health System in Philadelphia. He is the author of To Treat or Not To Treat and Death With Dignity and has published numerous peer-reviewed articles in national and international medical and ethical journals.

Contents

Preface

The field of Medical Ethics, also known as Bioethics, has grown exponentially over the years especially in its expertise and funding. If we date it back to the Seattle Artificial Kidney Selection Committee, also known as the "God Squad" in 1962, we understand that the field of Bioethics is about a half of century old. Bioethics has become established as an academic discipline with numerous journals and professional societies, it is reported on regularly in the media and its issues impact the lives of people globally. In developed countries, numerous political, social and economic developments have increased the number of ethics committees, Institutional Review Boards (IRBs) and ethics consults in general. In addition, academic programs for undergraduate and graduate students are increasing and flourishing. Global conferences on every conceivable medical-ethical issue are well attended by medical, ethical and legal colleagues and reported on extensively by the media. The prominence of bioethics has grown and continues to grow on a daily basis. With this growth come challenges. Academic bioethicists are challenged to teach about new issues like face transplants while showing how their analysis is based on previous related cases such as heart and hand transplants. Clinical bioethicists are confronted with financial and resource allocation issues that have a direct impact not only on patient's lives but on hospitals as well. Internationally, bioethicists are confronted by first world researchers and sponsors dedicated to overcoming various diseases but who fail to examine pertinent ethical issues that have a direct impact on human subject research. Sponsors of international research follow the spirit of international guidelines but often fail to follow the letter of the law that grounds these guidelines to protect human subjects in-country and provide sustainable benefits to in-country residents. Resources necessary to provide basic care to patients such as adequate pain management for cancer patients are available in abundance in developed countries but are lacking miserably in developing countries. Patients in many developing countries are sent home withering in pain with nothing more than ibuprofen to control their pain. These patients die horrible deaths and lack the basic dignity and respect that all human persons deserve. What has become a medical standard of care in many First World countries is limited by resources and injustices in many Third World countries. These profound limitations have become topics of concern for many international Bioethics societies and conferences.

The strength of this book on contemporary issues in bioethics is that it examines many of the critical medical-ethics issues that confront all of us today. Bioethics has become the business of everyone because it touches the lives of everyone. The ethical implications of issues like genetic engineering, genetic therapy, physician-assisted suicide, nanotechnology, reproductive technologies, stem cell research, cloning, end-of-life issues, organ transplantation, and health care reform go beyond individual hospitals, research centers and nursing homes. How these issues are resolved will determine for years and even decades who we are, not only as individuals, but who we are as a global community. These issues need to be examined broadly by individuals of varying talents, because these issues are far too important and life-changing to be left in the hands of a few medical professionals and researchers. The main strength of this book is that this international exchange of ideas will not only highlight many of these crucial issues but will strengthen the discipline of bioethics globally. A critical exchange of ideas allows everyone to learn and benefit from the insights gained through others' experiences. Analyzing and understanding real bioethics issues and cases and how they are resolved is the basis of education in bioethics for those who will have to make these decisions in the future. The more we examine, analyze, and debate these bioethics issues and cases, the more knowledge will be gained and hopefully, we will all gain more practical wisdom for the benefit of humankind.

Peter A. Clark
Director-Institute of Catholic Bioethics,
Saint Joseph's University,
Philadelphia, Pennsylvania,
USA

Dedication

I dedicate this book to my sister and brother-in-law, Mary Beth and Dominic Moffa and my nephews and niece, Nicholas, Andrew and Michelle Moffa, for instilling in me their love and knowledge and their courage to question.

1

Two Cautions for a Common Morality Debate: Investigating the Argument from Empirical Evidence Through the Comparative Cultural Study Between Western Liberal Individualist Culture and East Asian Neo-Confucian Culture

Marvin J. H. Lee
Philadelphia,
USA

1. Introduction

What I aim at in this essay is to give a guideline to contemporary common morality debate, as I point out what I see as two common problems that occur in the field of comparative cultural studies related to the common morality debate. Since the issues about common morality become increasingly important in today's medical ethics, this paper would help, I hope, particularly medical professionals, medical ethicists, hospital lawyers, etc. The thesis of this paper is as follows. In the field of contemporary comparative cultural studies with regard to common-morality theses[1] and to opposing theses of common morality[2], so-called the

[1] Common morality can be viewed broadly in two ways. One is the descriptive sense of common morality, which takes morality broadly as the "morality commonly practised by rational people." The earliest use of this sense may be John Stuart Mill's "customary morality" in Ch. 3 *Utilitarianism*. In the contemporary bioethical discussion, the plainest version of the descriptive sense of common morality simply affirms the phenomenon that a vast majority of, not all, people agree about a set of moral precepts or codes. The other is the prescriptive or normative sense of common morality. Taken in this sense, it argues that people *ought to* obey a set of moral precepts or codes. However, in the contemporary bioethics field, not only the descriptive but also the prescriptive senses of common morality are discussed without being conceived necessarily as universal or absolute, in the sense that common morality does not need to apply to all people and all times. (Carson Strong, "Exploring Questions about Common Morality," *Theoretical Medicine and Bioethics* 30, no. 1 [January 2009]: 3). Therefore, in the common morality debate, the "grouping issue" - that is, drawing the line by a region, a timeline, a religion, a country, etc., to group people common morality applies to - is one of the most important topics. In this essay, I use the term "common-morality" to include the both the descriptive and prescriptive senses. Also, it should be noted that the argument by empirical evidence can be used either to affirm or to deny the both senses of common morality.

[2] A variety of opposing theories or theses of common morality are available. Some examples are as follows. Isaiah Berlin's value pluralism, though it is a metaethical rather than normative theory, argues that certain moral values are equally valid and fundamental but incompatible with each other ("incompatible" in the sense that they can be in conflict with each other) and however that there cannot be a lexical ordering of these incompatible values (thereby making themselves "incommensurable" to

"argument from empirical evidence" has been the most popular argument. The opponents of common morality have presented the examples that show how the cultures in question differ from each other in their respective moral judgments or evaluations. On the other hand, the defenders of common morality have stressed homogeneity between different cultures by adducing some selected examples of their own. However, I find both dissenting parties' arguments careless, if not misleading, for two reasons. I lay out the reasons under the title of "two cautions" the both parties need to have when they argue. First, the advocates of and the opponents of common morality, I observe, consciously or unconsciously, fabricate the definitions of moral terms that would naturally lead to the outcomes they desire. To elaborate it in detail, I use two levels of understanding moral terms, that is, "formal level" and "material-content level." The formal level of understanding is to define the terms in a thin manner. The concept is thin in the sense that the meaning of the term is broad and general. On the other hand, the material-content level of understanding is to conceive the terms in a thick manner. The thick meaning is attained when people try to understand the terms against concrete situational contexts which involves rich cultural elements. The same moral term can be defined in the thin, formal level, as well as in the thick, material-content level. For example, "autonomy" can be understood in the formal level as "self-governed act," and in the material-content level as "the act of making their own informed decisions on their own life and death." The researchers of comparative cultural studies, of course, give at times a definition thinner than the former and thicker than the latter. The researchers devise the formal or material-content meanings of the moral terms in their own thickness or thinness level, the fact of which predetermines what examples they would select for their comparative cultural investigations and how they would interpret the examples to support their differing theoretical positions, either *pro* or *contra* common morality. However, given that the formal and material-content levels of understanding the terms are both theoretically valid and philosophically important, the backbone of their arguments from empirical evidences, i.e., that a set of neutral examples the researchers impartially discover in different cultures supports their theoretical conclusions, is defeated.

Second, the examples chosen to be the empirical evidences may not be as simple and clear-cut as the researchers think they are, mainly because the situational contexts where the cases are located between two different cultures vastly differ. Accordingly, the examples may not be proper to be "evidences." However, this does not support the opposing theses of common morality. Rather, it just shows that there are hardly "proper data", based on which two cultures can be compared.

To elaborate the thesis so far in organized details and to flesh it out in actual cases of comparative cultural studies, this paper has the following arrangement. The first two

---

each other). Religious-moral pluralism, a corollary of John Hick's religious pluralism, many see, argues that religious-moral diversities in the world point to metaphysical reality. Moral relativism (an orthodox kind) makes the prescriptive claim that there are no fixed "moral absolutes." Moral subjectivism typically starts with the claim (owing to David Hume) that moral evaluation/decision or the existence of moral concepts is merely the product of human mind; nevertheless, this position can depart from here to argue that the morality as what human mind creates embraces the fact that the fundamental moral structure of human beings is the same thereby producing similar, if not same, moral codes. However, when this subjectivism delimits its claim purely as descriptive, it can be an opposing view of the prescriptive sense of common morality.

following sections will be devoted to setting out the meanings of some key terms used in this paper. First, "culture" and "tradition" are defined. Second, the "formal level" of and "material-content level" of understanding moral terms are spelled out. In the following section, I provide general background of and some detailed content of two different cultures. I select Western liberal individualist culture and East Asian neo-Confucian culture. Since this paper intends to be presented to the audiences familiar with the liberal individualist culture, introducing its basic content and background is deemed unnecessary. Thus, neo-Confucian culture is only introduced. In the next section, against the backdrop of the knowledge provided so far, I show a set of examples of comparative culture between the Western and the East Asian culture. The cases will show how the different cultures respectively understand "beneficence" and "autonomy," the two concepts widely used in the field of medical ethics. Meanwhile, under the title of "two cautions," I attempt to show how different choices of defining the same moral terms by the researchers would influence their interpretations of the moral structure of the two cultures compared. In the conclusion section, I make my own suggestion where the current scholarly investigation of comparative cultural studies vis-à-vis common morality should be directed to, particularly from the perspective of contemporary medical ethics.

2. A traditon and a culture

Following Stephen Mulhall and Adam Swift's usage, I define the term "tradition" as the medium by which "a set of practices" "are shaped and transmitted across generations." It refers primarily to "religious or moral (e.g., Anabaptist or humanist), economic (e.g., a particular craft or profession, trade union or manufacturer), aesthetic (e.g., modes of literature or painting), or geographical (e.g., crystallizing around the history and culture of a particular house, village or region)."[3] I consider what is referred to as "culture" to hold the same meaning as the tradition, though the geographical boundary of the former should be broader than that of the latter. Along with the definitions above, I also propose "complimentary definitions" [4] of culture and tradition. That is, tradition and culture are essentially psycho-epistemic phenomena. Given that culture has a larger geographic boundary than tradition, the former can be said a macro psycho-epistemic phenomenon while the latter a micro one. And readers should note that what I want to treat in this paper is culture rather than tradition, i.e., Western liberal individualist culture and East Asian neo-Confucian culture.

A culture influences a tradition and vice versa. The former is the case, as the culture influences how people within its boundary should think and behave by determining social and ethical values in it. Thus, traditions that exist within the culture (if they are not extremely isolated ones like that of the Amish community) cannot be intact from the influence of the culture. On the other hand, the tradition can influence the culture. Traditions are destined to play by the rule of survival of the fittest within the boundary of the culture the traditions belong to, so the strong or powerful traditions continue to survive and thrive while participating in re-shaping of the culture. Having said so, I focus, in this essay, on power of culture, not tradition. Readers should note culture's power on the

[3] Stephen Mulhall and Adam Swift, *Liberals and Communitarians* (Oxford: Blackwell, 1992), 90.

[4] Note that two complementary meanings are two different, yet legitimate, ways of interpreting one and the same state of affair.

tradition. A good example of this can be to compare how Christian churches (or Christian traditions) within the contemporary Western liberal individualist culture, such as Britain and North America, celebrate St. Patrick's Day and Christmas, with how they did in the Medieval Europe.

3. Two different levels of understanding moral terms

The set of concepts like "form" and "material content" is widely used in ethics debates today. If the value, "do not lie", is a "formal" ethical injunction, its "material content" stipulates how to carry out the injunction in a concrete situational context. The material contents come in different shapes and sizes depending on the situational context. The formal principle, "do not lie", has various material contents, one of which can be "physicians must not withhold from their patients the information related to the patients' health condition." Some material contents are more specific than others. In many cases, the material content gets more specified as the scope and range of the value gets further elaborated. For instance, the material content introduced above can be further specified to "physicians must not withhold from their cancer patients the information that the patients will die soon." And a greatly specified material content appears, as the ethicist uses the "metaphor of specification" to solve moral dilemmas, particularly by using except- and unless-clauses.[5] E.g., the conflict or tension between "do not lie" and "save others" can be specified away by forming the following specified rule, "physicians must not withhold from their cancer patients the information that they will die *except-that* (or *unless*) it seems greatly obvious that the information revealed will harm the patients like increasing distress or shortening life significantly by shock."

To make clear how the form and material content are used as two different levels of understanding moral terms, another popular set of concepts used in contemporary ethics and bioethics should be introduced, that is, "thick" and "thin," the concepts known to be coined by Bernard Williams. In my expansion of Williams' terms, the "thick" and "thin" have at least two different sets of meanings. The first set is to understand the concepts in terms of a *theoretical status*. E.g., an ethical theory or principle or concept is "thick" in the sense that it treats practical moral life or is concerned with concrete/substantive level of morality; whereas "thin" in that it covers the abstract or speculative realm of morality. The other set is to conceive the thick and thin from the standpoint of *content*. E.g., the theory or principle or concept is "thick" in that it utilizes the values or norms or virtues that a particular culture or tradition holds, while "thin" in that it handles moral values or norms or virtues in a minimal sense.[6] In this essay, I shall focus only on the latter set, the "thick" and "thin" viewed in the light of content.

A moral term can have thick and thin definitions. To speak from the standpoint of comparative cultural studies, the thick definition of the term is the meaning attained as a particular society understands the term against its rich cultural backdrop. In other words, the thick definition has a culture-specific meaning. On the other hand, the thin definition of

[5] For the except- and unless-clauses, see Paul Ramsey, "The Case of the Curious Exception" in *Norm and Context in Christian Ethics* (1968), 74-93.

[6] It should be noted that the two ways of using the terms sometimes overlap.

the term is minimal in that its meaning is attained when people try to understand the term in a broad and general sense. Thus, the thin definition is mostly cross-cultural. However, the thick and thin definitions are not absolute or in isolation; they are in gradation and relative to each other. That is, the less thick the definition is, the thinner it is.

These definitions are not obtained through a neutral scholarly observation. How thinner or thicker the definition can be is determined based on how detailed the researchers go down to define the word in terms of including culture-specific materials. For example, defining the Korean moral term, *han*, has been one of the most interesting projects in the community of East Asian Christian theologians. Some scholars claim that *han* is so unique that it cannot be translated into the term which Westerners can grasp. For example, the Korean theologian, Jae Hoon Lee defines *han* to be something like "frustrated wish," "depressed anxiety," "envy," etc. stored deep in Korean mind through their unique cultural history as oppressed people.[7] He finds the uniqueness of *han* to lie in the Korean culture shown in "art, music, dance, and paintings . . . and literature (like poetry, folktales, myths, legends, novels, and theater)."[8] In sum, he views *han* in the thick definition. On the other hand, some theologians, like Andrew Sung Park, argue that the meaning of *han* is accessible to all cultures. For Park, the meaning of *han* is rather cross-cultural, in the sense that all cultures can understand it in a universal theological program. For him, *han* is "anger and bitterness of victims," while sin is "willful harm done to others." Hoping to improve what he believes to be one sidedness of the traditional Western doctrine that focuses on "sin," Park argues that the concept of *han* should be accepted as parallel to sin in the Christian theology. If sin is the problem on the side of the oppressor, *han* is that on the side of the oppressed, he claims. In short, Park sees the meaning of *han* in the thin definition.[9]

To return to the discussion of form and material content, the thin definition, as readers may already have noticed it, concerns the formal understanding of the term, while the thick definition largely bears the material content of the formal conception of the term. To put alternatively, inasmuch as comparative cultural study is concerned, the formal level of understanding of the moral term is to conceive the term to be thin, that is, minimal, general, and cross-cultural; while the material-content level of understanding is to view the term as thick, that is, culture-specific. If so, for instance, to conceive "honesty" and "beneficence" as thin definitions (respectively to be the "act of telling truth" and to be a "charitable act") is to understand the terms in the formal level. However, two different cultures may differ when their respective members understand what the acts are in terms of material content. E.g., North Koreans may apprehend the charitable act as related to obeying the will of their beloved leader, Kim Jŏng-il, whereas many North Americans and Western Europeans understand the charitable act to include endorsing women's right on abortion and gay marriage. To define autonomy and beneficence while being sensitive to cultural variation is to understand the terms to be thick as well as be in the material-content level. I believe I can turn now to comparative cultural studies.

---

[7] Jae Hoon Lee, *The Exploration of the Inner Wounds – Han* (Atlanta, Georgia: Scholars Press: 1994) 14, 33, 52. Note that *han* is not always a collective term. It can be for a group or an individual.

[8] Ibid., 1-2. For understanding of *han* in terms of its cultural uniqueness, see chapter 5, "The Han in the Symbolism of Korean Shamanism."

[9] Andrew Park, *The Wounded Heart of God* (Nashville: Abingdon Press, 1993), 10.

4. A short introduction to neo-Confucian ethics in Korean society

I begin with the general background and content of neo-Confucianism in Korea (South Korea). Initially, Confucianism as a fragmented set of Confucian tenets may have reached the Korean peninsula through the Chinese officials who dominated the northern part of Korea during the first three centuries A.D. It is reportedly said that in A.D. 372 a Confucian academy was established in the ancient Korean kingdom, Koguryŏ (B.C.37-A.D.668). However, it was not until the rise of the Chosŏn dynasty in the 14th century that Korea officially transformed itself into a Confucian kingdom. The new dynasty set out by adopting the Chinese philosopher, Zhu Xi's version of Confucianism (which we usually call "neo-Confucianism") as the nation's ethico-political ideology as well as practical governing principles.[10] Since then, neo-Confucianism has been one of the most powerful intellectual elements consisting of Korea's social and ethical milieu.

To discuss the practical ethical ethos of neo-Confucian East Asia (particularly Korea), it seems apt to introduce the ethical codes of the "Three Bonds and Five Relations" (三綱五倫) - note that the "bond" here means not merely a relationship but a standard. The Three Bonds state that the cosmic, *a priori* moral bonds are hierarchically set as 1) the son loves and serves his father (父爲子綱), 2) the subject loves and serves his king (君爲臣綱), and 3) the wife loves and serves her husband (夫爲婦綱). In accordance of the cosmic statutes, the Five Relations stipulate the presence of 1) trust and faith or *yi* (義) between king and subject (君臣有義), 2) filial-parental affection or *qin/chin* (親)[11] between father and son (父子有 親), 3) a distinction or *bie/byul* (別) between husband and wife (夫婦有別), 4) an order or *xu/suh* (序) between the older and the younger (長幼有序), and 5) loyalty or *xin/shin* (信) between friends (朋友有信).[12] As shown, the first four relations hold hierarchical structures and the last non-hierarchical one.

Many scholars believe that the Three Bonds and Five Relations were propagated by the Chinese philosopher and politician, Tung Chung-chu. Tung, as a chief minister to the emperor Wu (c. 140-87) of the Chinese Han dynasty, was responsible for the dismissal of all non-Confucian scholars from government and merging the Confucian and Yin-Yang schools of thought. Due to him, Confucianism (or neo-Confucianism) became the unifying ideology of the Han dynasty.[13] In fact, this endeavor of Master Tung reflects one of the core features of neo-Confucianism. No matter how speculative and theoretical issues Confucian scholars engage in, and though the scholars different metaphysical stances sometimes lead to the formation of unpleasant political factions, the ultimate philosophical aim they must pursue

---

[10] Martina Deuchler, *The Confucian Transformation of Korea: A Study of Society and Ideology* (Cambridge, MA: Harvard University Press, 1992), 14-27. Cf. for a rather detailed account of how the Chosŏn dynasty set out as a Confucian nation, see "The Ideology of Reform," chapter 6 of John B. Duncan, *The Origins of the Chosŏn Dynasty* (Seattle: University of Washington Press, 2000), and also Chai-sik Chung, "Chŏng Tojŏn: 'Architect' of Yi Dynasty Government and Ideology," in *The Rise of Neo-Confucianism in Korea*, ed. Bloom, Chan and de Bary, *Neo-Confucian Studies* (New York: Columbia University Press, 1985).

[11] *Qin* is how 親 pronounced in Chinese and *chin* is in Korean; and this order of Chinese/Korean pronunciation is henceforth maintained.

[12] All translations so far are mine.

[13] Wing-tsit Chan, "Yin Yang Confucianism: Tung Chung-Chu," in *A Source Book in Chinese Philosophy*, ed. Wing-Tsit Chan (Princeton, NJ: Princeton University Press, 1963, 1973), 271-273, 277.

is "to promote good character, dispositions, and consequent good actions."[14] In other words, in neo-Confucianism, *metaphysics is in service of ethics*. Accordingly, the Confucian governments naturally have had the perennial interest of inculcating moral virtues to the unlettered masses. For this reason, the Three Bonds and Five Relations, as the government's politico-ethical project, were constantly preached and upheld to moralize the members of the society in the Moral Way, which they believed is the (neo-) Confucian way.[15]

In Korea, the spreading of the Three Bonds and Five Relations, many scholars find, largely has to do with the work of Chŏng Yakyong (pen name Tasan, 1762-1834). As a high government official and an influential scholar in the late Chosŏn dynasty, Tasan proposed the most practical interpretation of the theory of Zhu Xi, the founder of neo-Confucianism. Tasan as leader of *Silhak* movement (the movement of practical scholarship) understood human nature not from the metaphysical but from the psychological sphere and observed the nature itself to be neither good nor evil but to be "potentially good" in that the exercise of free will in a right way makes the human nature better.[16] For him, the right moral path of exercising the free will is to develop the only true virtue, which he identifies as benevolence or love or humanity or *jen/in* (仁).[17] For him, *jen* is the collective or generic name for the three essential virtues that sustain right human relationship, i.e., filial piety or *xiao/hyo* (孝), fraternal respect or *ti/che* (悌), and compassion or *ci/cha* (慈).[18] The supreme virtue of *jen*, he asserts, is "symbol for the number two" because it is "the association for two people."[19] E.g., one meets another or others in a two-people relation. If I treat my elder brother with fraternal respect or *ti*, it is *jen*. If I serve my king with loyalty, it is *jen*. Also, "the fulfillment of respective duties in relationship between all pairs of people, including spouses and friends, is *jen*." With all these, Tasan could argue that the three virtues are equated with the Five Relations.[20] In other words, for him, the Five Relations are normative ethical directives inherently laden with the three virtues.

Neo-Confucian ethics presupposes the *a priori* moral path, based upon which all human beings are closely and rightly related to one another, and sees the society as a grand family where all members in it are bonded to one another as fathers/mothers, sons/daughters, older brothers/sisters, younger brothers/sisters, etc. Thus, maintaining and strengthening the "right kind of interpersonal relationship" - e.g., caring-parents and obeying children, caring husbands and respecting wives, caring teachers and submissive students, caring physicians and the patients that put great trust and respect in the physicians, etc. - is the

---

14 John Berthrong, "Dead Riders and Living Horses: The Problem of Principle/*Li* 理," in *International Conference on the Development of the Worldviews in Early Modern Asia* (Center for the Study of East Asian Civilizations at National Taiwan University: 2005), 4.

15 Peter H. Lee, "Versions of the Self," in *The Rise of Neo-Confucianism in Korea*, ed. Irene Bloom, Wing-tsit Chan, and Wm Theodore de Bary (New York: Columbia University Press, 1985), 484.

16 Mark Setton, "Tasan's 'Practical Learning'," *Philosophy of East and West* 39, no. 4 (Oct. 1989): 380.

17 "仁" is pronounced *jen* in Chinese and *in* in Korean. This order of marking is maintained throughout this essay.

18 Setton, "Tasan's 'Practical Learning,'" 382-386.

19 In fact, the Chinese character "仁" *jen/chen* pictographicallyis represents the relationship between "two people." For further discussion, see Judith A. Berling, "Confucianism," *Asian Religions* 2, no. 1 (Fall 1996), p.5.

20 Setton, "Tasan's 'Practical Learning'."

center of neo-Confucian practical ethics. In this sense, neo-Confucian ethics is in some way a more developed variation of the Western care ethics and some postmodern ethics. In Korean context, Tasan's unique rendering of the Three Bonds and Five Relations as the practical ethical codes in which the ideals of cosmic Confucian moral virtues are embodied is one important example that shows how serious Korean scholar-politicians were when they attempted to shape the practical moral mentality of their countrymen in accordance with the Confucian Path.

Over the last century until now, as part of modernization, the Western power has caused ideological, political, and economic shifts in Korea, particularly in urban areas. Nevertheless, many scholars find contemporary South Korea to be the model in which the most successful settlement of Confucian/neo-Confucian ideology is found. In South Korea, it is fairly easy to see the Confucian influence in every corner of the country. Older people are greatly respected. Even slight differences in ages are acknowledged. The proper sense of "friendship" exists only between the same age people. Even a one-year difference in age makes two people in a hierarchical relationship; the younger person is expected to call the older person "older brother/sister," not by his/her first name. Among a group of friends or co-workers, the oldest person is expected to pay in a restaurant or bar and the youngest is expected to pour wine or beer and serve the food. Differences in social ranks are also recognized; the relationship between juniors and seniors (in the order of rank) in social institutions (e.g., private companies, militaries, government offices, etc.) is highly important. The juniors are supposed to obey the seniors with the same kind of respect they give to their older brothers and sisters and their parents, and the seniors are to take care of the juniors with the same sort of affection they give to their younger brothers and sisters and their children. A family plays a very special role in the society. For Koreans, family is not only the bond that the Heaven ties in an individual level but also the conservatory of social morality. The family feels corporate responsibility for its member when the member violates social norms. Also, defying one's own parents, particularly the father, is considered a hideous act, the act blamable by the entire society.

5. Two cautions

I have so far, in a brief fashion, tried to account for what neo-Confucianism is, largely from the standpoint of practical/social ethics, and show how the Confucian ethical ideology appears in everyday life of contemporary South Korea. In this section, I want to focus on two particular moral values, "autonomy" and "beneficence," and attempt to show how the researchers' different choices of interpreting the same moral terms influence their own understandings of the moral structure of different cultures compared, insofar as common morality is concerned.

First, let us say that "beneficence" is defined as "charitable act or state," and "autonomy" "self-governed act or state." Defining the terms in this thin manner is a way of understanding them in a formal level. Both members of the liberal individualist and neo-Confucian cultures should feel the definitions valid. The lexical definitions of the words in standard Korean language dictionaries, "자선 (beneficence)" and "자율 (autonomy)," also confirm the soundness of this formal way of understanding the terms. If so, it turns out that neo-Confucian and the liberal individualist cultures share the meanings of "beneficence" and "autonomy." Then, could the moral values be in tension or in conflict with each other in certain situations?

To begin, it is interesting to note that neo-Confucianism's emphasis on "the senior's care for juniors"[21] and "the junior's respect for seniors" has resulted coincidently in uplifting the Hippocratic paternalism as a great moral value in hospitals in Korea - it is to be reminded that the terms "senior" and "junior" here are used in reference to both age and rank in social institutions. For Koreans, the doctor's beneficence that the Hippocratic paternalism stresses is regarded as the value of the senior's care for juniors that the Confucianism promotes, given that the medical doctors in Korea is treated like a Confucian elder due to their respected social position. Accordingly, in Korea, patients in general are not likely to challenge what their doctors recommend the patients should do. It is the fact that the Korean doctors' medical advises carry more weights to their patients than those of the Western doctors to their patients, and that the patients' trust and respect for their doctors are greater in Korea than in North American and Western Europe. In Korean soap-operas, movies, documentaries, the oft-used "moving scenes" are that the spouses or parents of terminally ill patients literally bow their heads down to the feet of their doctors, asking for help.[22] In this cultural atmosphere, "beneficence" as the doctor's charitable act is taken into much more serious consideration than "autonomy" as the patient's self-governed act. This contrasts with the fact that the Hippocratic paternalism has largely been evicted from many Western countries and is sometimes considered even a moral disvalue or a form of patronization, as liberal individualism has dominated the Western cultural ethos.[23] Note that Daniel Callahan observes and says that, due to the cultural/traditional dominance of liberal individualism in the West, moral solution of many Western ethicists, like the principlists, Tom Beauchamp and James Childress, always ends in giving priority to autonomy over beneficence.[24]

Despite all these, however, it is highly difficult to say that beneficence is prioritized over autonomy in Korea. If we ask any Koreans whether the doctor's charitable act is considered weightier than the patient's self-governed will or vice versa, without raising a particular case of conflict or tension between the two values in detail, most of them may answer that the patient's will should be considered first because, bluntly put, "decisions on your own health, or on your own life or death are ultimately your own business, though doctors' words should be respected." Besides, as it is the case in the Western countries as well as in Korea, actual moral verdicts in hospital seem de-facto legal ones, in that the cases are solved in the way that the doctors, nurses, and hospital lawyers may not legally be liable for the final agreements they come to with the patients and their families. Because of that, the actual

[21] Unlike in the Western societies, the "care for senior citizens" is a derogatory term in the Confucian East; it must be (the younger people's) "respect to senior citizens."

[22] This is more prevalent in the working class than the upper class people and in suburban than urban areas. In urban areas and for the upper-high class, individualism alongside the Western capitalistic lifestyle has been expanding.

[23] Perhaps, the majority of people in both cultures are short of the proper understandings of the Hippocratic texts. To read the texts properly, we may need an appreciation of the nuances of social relations and expectations.

[24] Daniel Callahan, "Principlism and Communitarianism," *Journal of Medical Ethics* 29, no. 5 (2003): 288-289.

cases in Korean hospitals turn out in the way that the will of the patients is granted through their own expressions, advance directives, or surrogate autonomy.

Here, the advocates of common morality can argue as follows. The denizens of neo-Confucian and the liberal individualist cultures both recognize and share the meanings of "beneficence" and "autonomy" respectively as the "charitable act" and as the "self-governed will." Also, both cultures prioritize autonomy over beneficence, they may emphasize, *in general*, in the sense that both cultures agree with the prioritization without getting involved with particular cases in detail. If so, they can argue, it can be said that, at least in a weak sense, both cultures consider autonomy weightier than beneficence, whereby giving to the validity of the existence of common, universal morality.

However, there is a way that the opponents of common morality can turn around the whole case in their favor. It is to investigate the cultures in a concrete, situational context. First of all, pointing out that the moral verdicts of actual cases in hospital may be all legal *de facto*, they can ask to put them aside and say that we need to discuss what is clearly moral in a hand-on level. Then, they can suggest that we better focus on how people in two different cultures understand moral terms on a concrete level. They may give beneficence and autonomy respectively the meanings of the "act of concealing from the terminally ill patients the information that they will die soon because it is likely that the information revealed will harm the patients like increasing distress or shortening life significantly by shock" and of "the act of making their own informed decisions on their own life and death."

I believe that the thick definitions like above are extremely proper in the Western hospital setting and well explain how people in the Western world (not only the Western liberal individualist world) think. From Judao-Christian Europe through modern and post-modern eras to contemporary liberal individualist period, the "human person" as a moral agent has been portrayed as a lonely being destined to seek one's own moral perfection, thereby being responsible for success or failure in one's own ethical journey. In short, a human person is an independent, if not isolated, being. Due to that, autonomy is the act of *my own* and beneficence that of *others*. Thus, it is natural that the meanings of beneficence and autonomy, whether thick or thin, are to be in conflict or in tension with each other.

However, that is not the case in neo-Confucian culture. Although thin, formal definitions of beneficence and autonomy may be in conflict or tension, the terms understood in a thick, material-content level are not to be in conflict or in tension. As mentioned earlier, the Confucian culture binds every individual in the society to be a member of the grand family. Thus, the neo-Confucian conception of a human person as an individual being is very different from the liberal individualist understanding of it. For Confucians, the human person is not an independent being but the one inherently dependent upon and personal to others within the web of society-family. Thus, in contrast to the liberal individualist view that "caring others" is my own act done to others whose ethical existence is ultimately independent from me, the Confucians regard "caring others" as my brotherly or sisterly act done to my own family members in a larger scale. In Korea it is customary that the terms like "father" "brother" "grandmother" "uncle" are used when complete strangers speak to one another. In retail stores, a female customer calls a female sales attendant "sister." A doctor in hospital calls his elderly patient "father" or "grandfather." A little schoolboy in the street calls an adult passerby "uncle" when he asks for direction. In this social atmosphere, proper interpretations of beneficence and autonomy in a concrete context must be in conjunction with an interpersonal relationship between a particular patient and the patient's doctor. If so, the two terms conceived in the thick level cannot have neat and isolated meanings to be compared, and thus not in conflict or in tension. The account so far will be more intelligent when rephrased through some particular cases.

Suppose that in Korea a 5-year-old child is terminally ill, her parents are about 30 years old, and the doctor in charge is about 50 years old. The parents feel morally bound to respect the doctor's decision. Even though the doctor's decision turns out later seriously mistaken, the parents would feel morally wrong to take a legal action against him (unless the doctor's decision is found to be out of his negligence or malintent). In analysis, the doctor's beneficence will be something like "the act of taking care of his young patient as if the patient were his own grandson, while incorporating the wishes of the child's biological parents as though they were the words of his own son or nephew or niece"; and that of the patient's autonomy is "the act of showing the patients' own wishes though his surrogate authority while taking into serious consideration of the doctor's advices as if they were their own father or uncle's words."

To give another example, suppose that a 60-year-old terminally ill patient's primary doctor is about 40 years old. Then, it is considered morally right that the doctor's beneficence must be expressed in the manner of filial piety towards the father-like patient. Note that in Korea it is very much common in hospitals that younger doctors and nurses call elderly patients "father," "mother," "grandfather," "grandmother," "uncle," "aunt," etc. Thus, the doctor's beneficence will be "the act of caring for his patient as if he were his own father or uncle." On the other hand, the patient cannot treat the doctor like his own child based on his seniority by age. As mentioned above, in neo-Confucianism, the authority of seniority is recognized by age and also by social rank. The medical doctors in Korea are treated like Confucian elders due to their respected social position. Hence, the patient's autonomy here will be like "the act of showing his own opinions while respecting the doctor's advices like his own father or uncle's words (by social rank)."

Due to the cultural atmosphere where everyone is considered a member of society-family, the meanings of two terms are laid out in conjunction or mixture with other moral values (e.g., care, respect, trust, etc.). Accordingly, their meanings are viewed organically intertwined rather than in conflict or tension.[25] Therefore, it is not only that beneficence and autonomy defined in the thick level cannot be in conflict or in tension, but also that the question whether beneficence is prioritized over autonomy does not arise - this fact, I believe, is one of the major reasons that normative practical ethics cannot come out of the Confucian East Asia.[26]

---

[25] Note the contrast with the Western liberal individualist culture where the meanings of beneficence and autonomy, thick or thick, are conceived mostly independently of other values.

[26] Despite my presentation has treated the cases of comparative cultures so far, the problem of language is not less serious within one culture. For example, beneficence and autonomy are not always in tension with each other, even in the Western liberal individualist ethics. E.g., the doctor's telling the patient about his terminally ill condition, in many cases, is taken to respect the patient's autonomy, which is in harmony with beneficence (allowing the patient to have relatively quality time without the fear of his

The great cultural difference exhibited, so far, through the cases of how the moral terms, beneficence and autonomy, are interpreted and used in the two different cultures, can give the opponents of common morality a firm ground to deny common-morality theses.

So far, I have tried to present the cases of comparative cultural studies in favor respectively of the advocates and the opponents of common morality, and to show that the forces of their arguments depend on how they define the moral terms they would like to use to investigate the cultures in question. The thinner definitions they use, it turns out, the more likely the defenders of common morality are to successfully argue for the validity of their thesis. And the thicker meanings they adopt, the more easily the opponents of common morality are to win the fight. Then, our question is which level of defining the terms, thick or thin, is valid or philosophically more important. I would say both levels are equally valid and important. The thin, formal level is almost identical to the usage of a standard language dictionary. As one of the important purposes of dictionary is, this broad way of understanding terms helps us conceptualize aspects of morality in an orderly manner. It's like filing data in our mind to understand what morality is. And what is amazing is that, regardless of cultural and traditional differences, we all understand and share this universal way of filing things and recognize its importance. On the other hand, the thick, material-content level of understanding moral terms is important in the way that we can understand how the terms are actually used in a particular context. As a result, it can be said that the arguments of both dissenting parties, the advocates and opponents of common morality, are consistent in their own constructs. However, given that the way they define the terms predetermines what they are going to argue, the kernel of their arguments from empirical evidence, that is, that a set of neutral examples the researchers impartially discover in different cultures supports their theoretical conclusions, is defeated.

The second caution I want to call for, though related to the first caution, is that the situational contexts where the cases of comparative culture are located are different, sometimes vastly different. In reality, the cases I presented above are usually entangled with more complicated interpersonal relationship. In the former case, for example, the 5-year-old patient might have 60-year-old grandparents and they might insist on their opinions on the child's condition against the doctor's will. Then, the case becomes the one we need to consider the values of the grandparents' beneficence/care for the child along with their senior authority, of the doctor's competing beneficence for the child with senior authority, and of the child's parents' respect for the two opposing wills between their parents and the doctor. Therefore, it is extremely difficult to locate any examples to be what the researchers call the "evidences." The evidences to be compared should be relatively simple and straightforward in the sense that the two cases compared have similitude in a large part and dissimilitude in some minor part. E.g., there can be good comparisons between baseball and softball, but not between baseball and canoeing. In other words, the example they find in one culture may not have its proper counterpart-example to be compared in another culture. However, this is not to say that the complexity that makes two cultures incomparable is a

soon-to-be-coming death). For many patients who put the value of autonomous decisions on their own lives over that of not having the fear of death, beneficence and autonomy collapse. I am grateful for Prof. Michael Langford at Cambridge for his comment here in the footnote.

premise in favor of the opposing thesis of common morality. It is just that there can hardly be "proper data", based on which two cultures can be compared, in order either to support or to deny common-morality theses.

6. Conclusion

The researchers of comparative cultural studies, I suggest, should be mindful of two things. First, there are two different levels of conceiving moral terms, i.e., formal and material-content levels, though the levels can only be understood in gradation from being thin to thick. And the researchers' pre-choice of how much thin or thick the meanings of the moral terms should be determines the conclusions they desire to support. This fact belies their held position of the argument from empirical evidences, namely, that a set of impartial discoveries as neutral evidences yields a conclusion, either *pro* or *contra* common-morality theses. Second, the complexity constituted out of the variety of situational contexts that different cultural ideologies produce is so great that the examples the researchers find in one culture may be unique to that particular culture, the fact of which makes comparative cultural investigation itself extremely difficult.

The argument from empirical evidences may be a myth. In comparative cultural study with regard to common morality, there should be a discussion whether or not the researchers can agree on or concede to a particular level of defining moral terms before delving into sets of examples to be found in different cultures. The agreement or concession can be philosophical (theoretical) or practical. The philosophical agreement on or concession to the particular level naturally yields to that of the position either of advocating or denying common-morality theses, while the practical agreement or concession does not. The practical agreement or concession has freedom of not binding itself to any one theoretical position. For this, critics may say that the agreement or concession out of practical reasons is making its validity based not on the higher standard of truths but on usefulness or practicality.[27] They may call the practical agreement or concession "utilitarian" in a nefarious sense. The critics are right that the practical reasons are not the higher standard of truths. However, I believe in as much as the reasons are balanced and in service of public good (good of a particular culture or tradition), they are good enough for us, particularly in the field of medical ethics.[28]

7. References

Beauchamp, Tom and James Childress. *Principles of Biomedical Ethics* (6th ed.). New York: Oxford University, 2009.

Berling, Judith A. "Confucianism." *Asian Religions* 2, no. 1 (Fall 1996): 5-7.

---

[27]Ana Iltis criticizes contemporary bioethics for being groundless or for making its validity based not on the higher standard of truths but on usefulness or practicality, etc. (Ana Iltis, "Bioethics as Methodological Case Resolution," *Journal of Medicine and Philosophy* 25 no. 3 [2000]: 278).

[28] As common morality advocates, Beauchamp and Childress argue that a good practical method based on common morality cannot buy into a full-blown theory primarily because there would not be a theory that can fully explain our common and diverse moral experiences. (Beauchamp and Childress, *Principles of Bioethical Medicine* 6th ed. [Oxford: New York 2009], 363-363)

Berthrong, John. "Dead Riders and Living Horses: The Problem of Principle/*Li* 理." In *International Conference on the Development of the Worldviews in Early Modern Asia*, 1-17. Center for the Study of East Asian Civilizations at National Taiwan University, 2005.

Callahan, Daniel. "Principlism and Communitarianism." *Journal of Medical Ethics* 29, no. 5 (2003).

Chan, Wing-tsit. "Yin Yang Confucianism: Tung Chung-Chu." In *A Source Book in Chinese Philosophy*, edited by Wing-Tsit Chan. Princeton, NJ: Princeton University Press, 1963, 1973.

Chung, Chai-sik. "Chŏng Tojŏn: 'Architect' of Yi Dynasty Government and Ideology." In *The Rise of Neo-Confucianism in Korea*, edited by Irene Bloom, Wing-tsit Chan and Wm Theodore de Bary, 59-88. New York: Columbia University Press, 1985.

Copi, Irving M., and Carl Cohen. *Introduction to Logic*. Edited by the 9th Edition. Englewood, New Jersey: Macmillan Publishing Company, 1990.

Deuchler, Martina. *The Confucian Transformation of Korea: A Study of Society and Ideology*. Cambridge, MA: Harvard University Press, 1992.

Duncan, John B. *The Origins of the Chosŏn Dynasty*. Seattle: University of Washington Press, 2000.

Iltis, Ana. "Bioethics as Methodological Case Resolution," *Journal of Medicine and Philosophy* 25 no. 3 (2000): 271-284.

Lee, Jae Hoon. The Exploration of the Inner Wounds – *Han*. Scholars Press: 1994, Atlanta, Georgia: Scholars Press, 1994.

Lee, Peter H. "Versions of the Self." In *The Rise of Neo-Confucianism in Korea*, edited by Irene Bloom, Wing-tsit Chan and Wm Theodore de Bary. New York: Columbia University Press, 1985.

MacIntyre, Alasdair. "Theology, Ethics, and the Ethics of Medicine and Health Care." *Journal of Medicine and Philosophy* 4, no. 4 (December 1979): 435-43.

Mulhall, Stephen, and Adam Swift. *Liberals and Communitarians*. Oxford: Blackwell, 1992.

Park, Andrew Sung. *The Wounded Heart of God*. Nashville: Abingdon Press, 1993.

Ramsey, Paul. "The Case of the Curious Exception." In *Norm and Context in Christian Ethics*, ed. by Gene Outka and Paul Ramsey. London, UK: Charles Scribner's Sons, 1968.

Setton, Mark. "Tasan's 'Practical Learning'." *Philosophy of East and West* 39, no. 4 (Oct. 1989): 377-92.

Strong, Carson. "Exploring Questions about Common Morality." *Theoretical Medicine and Bioethics* 30, no. 1 (January 2009): 1-9.

2

Ethical Resources for the Clinician: Principles, Values and Other Theories

Thomas M. Donaldson
University of Cambridge, UK

1. Introduction

Medical students heading out on to the wards can encounter a bewildering array of ethically problematic scenarios. A recent study (Donaldson et al., 2010) looking at how medical students define and discuss moral problems, identified a large number of issues as the source of these moral problems. These included situations involving decision making at the end of life, the termination of pregnancy, pre-natal testing, reproductive technologies, child protection issues, substance misuse, and interpersonal conflict. Many of these issues are focussed in or even unique to a medical setting, with little or no precedence or guidance available from life outside medicine. These were the issues that students raised, and they sought further ethical resourcing to guide them through these tricky situations.

Only a small percentage of the medical students had discussed their dilemma within an ethical framework, which may suggest a lack of knowledge of ethical theories to resource their thinking. However, some of the students used the Four Principles of medical ethics (Beauchamp and Childress, 2009) to analyse their cases, whilst others highlighted that conflict occurred as a result of a divergence in values. There were also students who discussed their cases in ways that suggested parallels with Kantian, Utilitarian and Virtue Ethics. These are all important ethical theories which form the basis of the resources available to clinicians facing such ethical dilemmas.

Ethics is the branch of philosophy striving to describe and discuss how to lead a good life and medical ethics is the application of ethics to the professional life of the clinician. This chapter will look in more detail at the key resources available from moral philosophy to the clinician faced with a medical ethical dilemma. Whilst full philosophical analysis of different theories is beyond the scope of this chapter, discussion of the strengths and weaknesses of the different resources from moral philosophy, when applied to a clinical setting, will allow suggestions to be made about how they can be useful to the clinician. The resources that will be covered are Principalism, Values Theory, Deontology, Teleology and Virtue Ethics.

2. The four principles (Beauchamp and Childress, 2009)

The Four Principles Approach to biomedical ethics (Principalism) put forward by Beauchamp and Childress is a tool for analysing ethical dilemmas using the principles of Beneficence, Non-Maleficence, Autonomy and Justice. These principles represent various traditions in ethical thinking and highlight different obligations and ideals. The weighing and balancing of these principles is suggested as a way to find a solution to ethical dilemmas. However, there is not clear guidance about how a clinician should weigh and balance the principles, and this is a limitation to the use of the Four Principles in a clinical setting.

2.1 Beneficence

The Principle of Beneficence refers to the moral imperative to act in such a way as to do good and benefit others. Beneficence arises from a number of traditions including Judeo-Christian ethics, the Hippocratic Oath as well as Utilitarianism, with its slogan "the greatest happiness for the greatest number," and the striving for good outcomes that is characteristic of Teleological Ethical Theories. The term Beneficence suggests acts of love, mercy, kindness and charity and this principle exhorts clinicians to act in a patient's best interests.

Beauchamp and Childress discuss to what extent Beneficence can be considered a moral obligation against which clinicians can be judged, rather than a moral ideal for clinicians to aspire towards. They conclude that there are some situations where Beneficence is obligatory, such as to family and those in close relationships, or scenarios where a significant good can be achieved, such as the rescue of a person in danger when there is no-one else closer and there is no significant danger to oneself. This obligation can extend to doctor-patient relationships.

The ideal of Beneficence, rather than Beneficence as an obligation, should be a powerful motivating factor for all clinicians. Every medical intervention offered to a patient should be done because of a belief that it will benefit the patient and out of a desire to do the patient good. Many clinicians have chosen this career out of a desire to use their professional life to do good for patients. Beneficence can thus be considered as the appropriate starting point with which to begin any analysis of a dilemma in medical ethics using the Four Principles, as the desire to do good for patients should be the motivation driving clinicians to seek the best resolution of the problem.

The other three principles of Non-Maleficence, Autonomy and Justice can be seen as principles that balance the beneficent desire of clinicians to do good for patients, in order to ensure that unrestrained and ill-considered good intentions do not lead to un-intended and potentially disastrous ethical outcomes.

2.2 Non-maleficence

The Principle of Non-Maleficence refers to the moral obligation not to inflict harm on others. This principle need not be limited to the prohibition of active harm but also implies an obligation not to expose patients to an increased risk of harm through negligence (whether intentional or not), departure from professional standards or a failure of a clinician's duty of care. Non-Maleficence is often ascribed to the Hippocratic tradition, although the often misquoted slogan "first do no harm" is not actually found in the Hippocratic Oath. However, Non-Maleficence is also an important feature of Deontological and Judeo-Christian ethical traditions.

Non-Maleficence acts as an important balance to the principle of Beneficence because no medical intervention is without risks or side effects, and all medical decision making involves a balancing of benefits and risks. The practice of medicine must not be overwhelmed by the desire to do good at any cost and the unchecked consideration of extra-ordinary or heroic treatments for patients could expose them to significant harms and risks for little potential benefit. For example, the balancing between Beneficence and Non-Maleficence is often important in decisions regarding managing patients at the end of life.

In such discussions the distinction between an act and an omission is an important one. The principle of Non-Maleficence implies a prohibition to clinicians acting in such a way as to harm patients, for example by administering potassium chloride to a patient with a terminal illness, even if the patient has requested this to end their suffering. However, the withholding or withdrawing of treatment by the clinician can be ethically viewed as an omission rather than an act, for example, the withdrawal of active treatment and the starting of palliative management for a patient with a terminal condition. The principle of Non-Maleficence should not be seen to prohibit such decisions. Instead the analysis of such a situation should be started with the principle of Beneficence, tempered and balanced by the principle of Non-Maleficence. A clinician should only provide a medical intervention if it is likely to benefit the patient, and so when it will no longer provide that benefit, such as to a patient with a terminal condition, then according to the principle of beneficence it can and should be withdrawn. Non-maleficence actually supports such a decision since the risks or side effects associated with any medical intervention could be harmful to a patient with a terminal condition and so should be avoided, especially if there is to be no benefit.

The principle of Non-Maleficence is not absolute and 'the Doctrine of Double Effect' is an example of a rationale for accepting that there are situations where a clinician can act in such a way which may result in harm to the patient, as long as the harm is not intended, but only foreseen. The main situation where 'the Doctrine of Double Effect' has been used is in the administration of analgesia in terminally ill patients with significant pain. In order to adequately control such pain it can be necessary to administer large doses of opiates, which risk the hastening of a patient's death. However, since this harm is not the intended consequence of the action, the intention is to control the pain, it is argued that this is ethically justifiable. Whilst 'the Doctrine of Double Effect' has proved a successful argument in the legal setting, it faces a number of philosophical challenges that are difficult to resolve. In particular it is difficult to provide a coherent and consistent account of what makes an outcome foreseen but not intended and yet another outcome foreseen and intended.

In complex situations arising from having two or more patients involved, the principle of Non-Maleficence can be difficult to apply. Kidney donors who undergo significant risks for no personal benefit are such an example. Non-Maleficence as an absolute principle would seem to prohibit such an intervention which can result in such a good outcome for another patient with renal failure. A pregnant woman who would die without a life saving treatment that would result in the death of her foetus demonstrates further difficulties, and the necessity of involving other principles, including those of Autonomy and Justice.

2.3 Respect for autonomy

Just as the principle of Non-Maleficence reminds the clinician not to intentionally harm a patient in their beneficent drive to do good, so the principle of Respect for Autonomy also balances Beneficence by posing the question: who decides what is good for the patient? Medicine has traditionally had a paternalistic ethos, with the expert clinician deciding for a patient what is best for them. Respect for Autonomy, however, is the principle that acknowledges the right of a patient to hold their own views and to make choices and take actions based on their particular views and beliefs. Autonomy has a strong base in Deontological ethics, Rights Theory and many Utilitarians also emphasise its importance. It is also the foundational principle in Values Based Medicine (which will be discussed later in the chapter).

Respect for Autonomy involves an obligation on the clinician not to control or constrain patients, and the importance of autonomous self-determination and bodily integrity necessitates that patient consent must be gained by a clinician proposing a medical intervention. This consent can be explicit consent (written or verbal) or implied/implicit consent. However in order to be valid, consent must be voluntary and informed. Therefore, respect for autonomy also imposes a positive obligation on the clinician to foster autonomous decision making, disclosing information and even striving to help patient's overcome unhealthy dependence on doctors. Respect for Autonomy involves both a respectful attitude towards patients as free individuals with their own legitimate values and beliefs, as well as respectful actions in providing information and facilitating decision-making to allow informed consent.

For Beauchamp and Childress, respect for Autonomy is a fundamental obligation for the clinician, rather than an ethical ideal to be strived for. However, the philosophical ideal of Autonomy in its purest sense of freedom from any form of influence is something that few (if any) patients are able to achieve. Nevertheless most patients can and do want to decide for themselves on the basis of their own beliefs and values (even if they are unable to express these values or they are not well thought out). There needs to be an excellent reason for overriding a patient's autonomous decision, and so the clinician's desire to do good for a patient should not override their autonomous refusal of their intervention. This has led to the concept of the "Autonomy trump card" or the "triumph of Autonomy", which demonstrate the power of the principle of Respect for Autonomy over other principles, especially in situations involving patients who are able to decide for themselves. Most of the time what the patient decides is what should happen.

There are, however, exceptions to the "Autonomy trump card", where concerns for Beneficence, Non-Maleficence and Justice can and do override patient autonomy. These tend to occur when a patient's decisions affect others, and the "greater good" must be considered. Such a situation is the notification of sexual partners of HIV affected patients, who could potentially be harmed by the patient's choice not to tell them this information. Another example is when public health is endangered, such as when an epileptic patient wants to choose to continue driving and the doctor may have a duty to prevent them doing so, for the greater good and to prevent harm to others. Also in situations where resources are scarce, a patient's choice may not actually be available to them, and considerations of Justice override Autonomy.

Not all patients are able to make autonomous decisions. Children, those suffering from acute attacks of certain mental illnesses, patients under the influence of strong drugs or otherwise incapacitated or unconscious are all often unable to make autonomous decisions. In treating such patients the concept of acting in their best interest (in line with the principle of Beneficence) becomes of vital importance. In order for a patient to be judged unable to make an autonomous decision their capacity (or competence) must be assessed. In order to demonstrate capacity to consent to treatment a patient must be able to understand the information needed to give informed consent, be able to retain it, be able to weigh and judge the information in light of their beliefs and values and be able to communicate their decision. Capacity is always specific to particular decisions or tasks, so whilst there may be certain decisions that a patient is not competent to make there may well be others things that they can decide for themselves. In addition, capacity may vary or be intermittent. Respect for Autonomy exhorts the clinician to strive to maximise a patient's capacity, by creating the best environment, optimising treatment and giving information in such a way as to allow patients to make decisions based on their own beliefs and values wherever possible.

Not all patients want to make autonomous decisions, and would rather ask their doctor to make a decision for them. Even though patients have the right to make decisions for themselves, this does not imply a duty upon them to do so. A patient's choice to delegate responsibility for a decision to their doctor is still an autonomous act.

2.4 Justice

The clinician who out of Beneficence would do good for his patient must weigh this good against the principle of Non-Maleficence and the principle of Respect for Autonomy. The final principle against which Beneficence must be weighed is that of Justice, which raises the issue of to whom the clinician should be doing good. This is vital to remember because a clinician and their patient, even in the privacy of a consultation room, are not alone in the world. Medicine is practiced in a world of great need and limited resources and it is important that the clinician should remember that, as well as the patient he is seeing today, there are many other potential patients who also have potential demands on medical resources. Why should the clinician treat one patient and not the other?

Theories of Justice arise from many ethical theories, and these describe Justice in very different ways. In Utilitarianism (which will be discussed later in the chapter) Justice is the same as utility, and as long as a situation has the best possible outcome it is deemed just, no matter what potential inequalities exist. Libertarian Theories see justice as fair process, so that a situation can be just even if outcomes are uneven, as long as individuals have had equal opportunity and so been subject to a just process. Justice in Egalitarian theories demands that persons should receive equal distribution of goods such as healthcare. However, it is also argued that not everyone should receive the same when the needs of different individuals vary. As Aristotle is quoted to have said, "equals should be treated equally, and unequals unequally".

The principle of Justice involves the allocation of resources, and different criteria have been proposed to guide this distribution. These include equal share, effort, contribution, merit, free market exchange and need. Beauchamp and Childress advocate distribution according to need. They also propose a fair opportunity rule, with distribution weighted to mitigate the negative effects of life's social and biological lotteries.

Beauchamp and Childress divide decisions of Justice into various categories. The first category of decisions are about how to allocate resources, such as political decisions of how much to allocate to a healthcare budget or how to allocate within health and healthcare budgets, all they way down to decisions regarding the allocation of scarce treatments to individual patients. The need for rationing creates another set of decisions of Justice. And finally the setting of priorities in healthcare also involves decisions of Justice. One of the key tools for this is cost-effectiveness analysis, which seeks to allow allocation of resources, rationing and setting of priorities in the most cost-effective way. One of the most important examples of such cost-effectiveness analysis are QALYs (quality adjusted life years). QALYs provide a measure of benefit weighted for quality of life and are an example of utilitarian calculus when applied to the question of Justice. QALYs will be discussed further later in the chapter.

The principle of Justice broadens the ethical responsibility of the clinician from the patient he is seeing and engages him in a world of medical need and limited resources. Peter Singer's Utilitarianism (Singer 1979) proposes a global perspective that every human has a right to a decent minimum of healthcare. Such an ethical demand can seem overwhelming and any individual clinician should obviously not feel responsible for providing complete global Justice. However, it is important for individual clinicians to remember that they are part of a healthcare response to a need that is global but whose resources are limited. The principle of Justice reminds the clinician that the good they intend to do for a patient must never be done out side of this wider context.

2.5 Strengths and weaknesses of the four principles

Principalism has been widely adopted in medical ethical thinking and education and there are many good reasons for this. The Four Principles are simple and easy to remember and yet provide a clinician with tools for ethical reasoning that arise from careful analysis, distillation and amalgamation of many theories and traditions of moral philosophy. The Four Principles are at their most useful to the clinician as concepts which allow the analysis of a decision or scenario from a number of different ethical perspectives. The perspectives of Beneficence, Non-Maleficence, Autonomy and Justice can provide insights into confusing situations and allow the reasons for this conflict to be clarified, as well as allowing reasoning and argument from different perspectives to be thoroughly examined.

The weakness of Principalism comes when the ethical analysis of a scenario is finished and a decision must be reached. Beauchamp and Childress suggest that the principles should be weighed against each other, but have been unable to offer a coherent account of how this should be done (De Grazia, 2003). There is no clear indication of when one principle should be deemed to be more important than another, and the most common default position is that Autonomy is given pre-eminence, though this is done without clear justification.

Donaldson et al's study of the cases brought by medical students for discussion in medical ethics seminars highlights this problem with Principalism. A number of the students used the Four Principles to analyse their case, but none of them had reached a conclusion through this process on what course of action should be taken. The hypothesis proposed as a result of the findings of this study suggested that the use of the Four Principles in medical ethics can lead medical students to see medical ethics as a discipline for analysing ethically problematic scenarios, without needing to reach a decision on the right course of action, and perhaps even leading to the belief that there is no right or wrong course of action (only legal or illegal ones).

A helpful method of weighing these principles against each other is to use Beneficence (the desire to do good) as the motivating drive for a clinician when faced with an ethical decision. This must then be weighed against Non-Maleficence, Autonomy and Justice

(Gillon 1985). If the ethical motivation to do good is not quenched or overridden by the perspectives of the other principles then this provides the clinician with an ethical justification for the intervention they propose. This method is by no means complete and does not answer the problem of specifying at what point one principle overrides another, and so the clinician may need to look to other ethical resources for guidance when faced with making an ethical decision and weighing between the principles.

As mentioned earlier, Teleological and Deontological ethics are both branches of moral philosophy that are important foundations for Principalism. Later in the chapter these philosophies will be discussed in more detail. Whilst it is beyond the scope of this chapter to give a full philosophical analysis of each theory, there will be discussion of each theory to unearth resources and insights that can be of use to the clinician who is balancing and weighing principles against each other. The chapter will also discuss virtue ethics, which has enjoyed a recent resurgence in moral philosophy, and offers a different perspective to resource the clinician. However, next for discussion is Values-Based Medicine.

3. Values-based medicine (Fulford, 2004)

Conflict was a recurring theme raised by medical students in cases brought for discussion in the study by Donaldson et al. It was hypothesised that the high frequency with which conflict was raised by medical students was because conflict is a good indicator that divergence of values has occurred. Values-Based Medicine is an approach to decision making in healthcare which emphasises the importance of acknowledging and exploring differences in values as part of the decision making process.

Values-Based Medicine is proposed as a counterpart to Evidence-Based Medicine. The progress of science has led not just to a growing complexity of facts (to which Evidence-Based Medicine is a response), but also to an increasing level of choice in the practice of medicine. Increasing choices, as well as an increasing diversity in society, contribute to an increasing complexity of values in the practice of medicine. The response proposed to this complexity by Bill Fulford is Values-Based Medicine and he outlines his theory in the 10 principles of Values-Based Medicine.

3.1 The 10 principles of values-based medicine

1. The "two feet" principle - The "two feet" on which all decisions stand are facts and values.
2. The "squeaky wheel" principle - Values, though present all the time, are most noticeable when different values conflict in decision making.
3. The "science-driven" principle - Scientific progress, far from making facts superior to values in decision making, increase the importance and diversity of values by creating a wider array of choices.
4. The "patient-perspective" principle - The perspective of the patient/patient group is of first importance in decision making
5. The "multiperspective" principle - Values-Based Medicine seeks to resolve conflicts of values through a process of balancing legitimately different perspectives, rather than by reference to a rule or "right outcome".
6. The "values-blindness" principle - Raising awareness of values is crucial to the practise of Values-Based Medicine, and careful attention to language is crucial to this.

7. The "values-myopia" principle - Values-Based Medicine encourages the clinician to improve their knowledge of values that may be held by other people, and that empirical and philosophical methods can be important resources for this.
8. The "space of values" principle - Values-Based Medicine uses ethical reasoning not to determine what is "right", but to explore differences in values as a resource to clinical decision making.
9. The "how it's done" principle - Communication and listening skills are central to Values-Based Medicine, both in establishing different values perspectives (especially the patient's perspective) and in resolving conflicting values to decide upon a practical course of action.
10. The "who-decides" principle - The importance of exploring and seeking to resolve differences in values makes decision making the job of clinicians and patients, rather than ethicists and lawyers.

3.2 Strengths and weaknesses of values-based medicine

Bill Fulford's assessment of the increasing complexity of both facts and values in medical practise, and his facts + values model of healthcare decision making are both hugely helpful insights. Values-Based Medicine also gives a very necessary challenge to clinicians to be aware of the potential for "value-blindness" and to seek to overcome or avoid this by making use of empirical and philosophical resources, as well as by focussing on the patient's perspective, the patient's narrative and the language that they use. In doing this, Values-Based Medicine adds to Bauchamp and Childress' principle of Autonomy, grounding what can otherwise be an abstract principle into clinical practice as well as equipping the clinician to negotiate their way through the complexities of clinical decision making whilst truly seeking to respect a patient's autonomy as they explore their values.

The focus on the skills, especially communication skills, required in healthcare decision making is also a valuable perspective that Value-Based Medicine brings to Medical Ethics. Reasoning and logic skills may suffice for the ethicist in an ivory tower, but will never be enough for a clinician making healthcare decisions in partnership with patients. Furthermore, that healthcare decision making should rightly happen in the clinical setting is another valuable insight of Values-Based Medicine. Values-Based Medicine also emphasises the importance of "right process" in healthcare decision making, rather than "right outcome". Whilst the importance of "right process" is often overlooked in medical ethics, right outcome cannot be neglected either. Both right process and right outcome are vital in healthcare decision making.

This leads into the main weakness of Values-Based Medicine, namely the inability to determine for a clinician what is right, even when they are fully aware and engaged with a patient's values. Values-Based Medicine is an analytical and descriptive tool that seeks to increase awareness and understanding of different values, rather than offering a resource to guide clinicians towards an understanding of the right decision, or even the right value. Values-Based Medicine also suffers from a similar criticism as Principalism, namely that of being useful in the analysis of ethical dilemmas or situations, but offering no definite guide to the right decision. However, whilst Principalism acknowledges the need to discover the right decision, Fulford's account of Values-Based Medicine criticises what he describes as the "quasi-legal model" of ethics which seeks for a "right" outcome and claims instead that different values should be seen as equal. Values-Based Medicine encourages clinicians not to judge or weigh values against each other, but rather it seeks to exhort the clinician to use communication skills to create a space in which values can co-exist. However, when directly opposing values are brought into conflict, the use of communication skills by the clinician to create such a space could seem to be little short of deception.

Even Fulford, in his account of the ten principles of Values-Based Medicine, acknowledges that not all values are equal, and only "legitimate values" (values legitimised by rules and regulation dictated by consensus of the community involved) should be included in healthcare decision making. In doing this, Fulford limits the scope of Values-Based Practice to a narrow range of decisions within tightly defined guidelines, and so seriously limits its usefulness to Medical Ethics. Values-Based Medicine cannot offer any explanation (beyond a mention of consensus, with no idea of how this could or should be reached) of the basis of these guidelines upon which it depends. Since the formation of such guidelines also falls into the remit of medical ethics, this is another aspect of the ethical endeavour for which Values-Based Medicine provides little or no resourcing. The usefulness of Values-Based Medicine is also limited by its inability to add anything to situations in medical ethics where a patient's values are not accessible to the clinician, such as in the treatment of either the child, the demented, the delirious, the intoxicated or the unconscious patient. Since these situations can be some of the most ethically difficult for the clinician, Values-Based Medicine cannot on its own provide a sufficient ethical resource. Values-Based Medicine is, therefore, best seen as a practical outworking of the principle of Autonomy. It can give clinicians skills and resources to understand a patient's perspective, but has little power to guide the clinician towards the right decision.

4. Teleological ethical theories

The term Teleological Ethics describes a group of theories that are focussed on the outcomes or consequences of actions, and so this group of theories are also described as Consequentialist Ethics. The word Teleology derives from the Greek word *telos*, meaning end or goal, and so Teleological Ethics regard an action as right or wrong according to the balance of good or bad consequences that it has. Therefore, the right act is the act with the best foreseeable overall result. According to Teleological Theories the only features of an act that are morally relevant are its foreseeable outcomes. The motivation for an action is, therefore, seen as irrelevant, as is the fact that an act may 'break the rules'.

In order for Teleological Ethics to be discussed as a complete moral theory it must give a valid account of what aspects of the consequences of actions are morally important. One answer to this suggestion comes from the most important of the Teleological Theories, Utilitarianism.

4.1 Utilitarianism (Bentham, 1789 and Mill 1861)

Whilst the ideas underlying Utilitarianism may stretch back as far as Epicurus, the fathers of Utilitarianism are Bentham and Mill, whose writings gave birth to the theory of Utilitarianism during the Enlightenment. They suggested that morality was not about faithfulness to a code or inflexible rules. Rather Utilitarianism is a monist theory, with one foundational principle against which the consequences of actions are to be judged. This principle is that of Utility – the "greatest happiness" principle, often captured in the slogan, "the greatest happiness for the greatest number". In Utilitarianism the overriding focus is the amount of happiness or unhappiness produced by an action.

Bentham argued that it is self evident that suffering is bad and happiness is good, and he saw suffering and happiness (described in terms of simple pleasure) as opposite poles of a continuum. From these intuitions he derived his hedonistic version of Utilitarianism, arguing that actions should be decided upon by determination of the net effects of potential alternative actions in terms of producing happiness or reducing suffering. The action that produces the most happiness, or the least suffering, is the right action. This is Bentham's hedonic calculus, which he proposed as a consistent and reliable procedure for making decisions. For Bentham, therefore, morality is the attempt to bring about as much net pleasure (pleasure minus suffering) as possible into the world.

Mill, however, gives an account of Utility that is not purely hedonistic, because his view of happiness is not based on simple pleasure. He argued that not all pleasures are comparable, and saw happiness in terms of eudaimonia (human flourishing, a concept that is important in virtue ethics and will be discussed later in greater detail). His famous quote, "better to be a human being dissatisfied than a pig satisfied", highlights this point. However, to Mill pleasure and pain are still fundamental to his understanding of happiness and his conception of Utility is still the balance of pleasure over pain.

Utilitarianism has been further developed by numerous philosophers. Modern liberal democracies have given rise to new concepts of Utility that emphasise the importance of maximising individuals' autonomous choices and preferences. This is seen as the best way of maximising happiness when people from diverse communities vary in their perceptions of happiness and flourishing. This approach also gives weight to the importance of Autonomy and the powerful desire for self determination that is a foundational principle of liberal democracies.

A further development of Utilitarianism is to move the place of Utilitarian calculus away from decisions about individual actions and use it instead in the formulation of rules, the following of which will maximise happiness and minimise suffering. This rule based application of utility to maximise welfare is described as Rule-Utilitarianism, to distinguish it from the Act-Utilitarianism of Bentham and Mill. Rule-Utilitarians will, therefore, argue that the rules should be obeyed even in situations where doing so may produce a negative outcome that will reduce the Utility. Their justification for this is the fact that the overall outcome of the rule still produces a net increase in Utility, even if it produces reduction in Utility in certain cases. However, it is possible to argue that this development of the Theory of Utilitarianism displays a lack of consistency from the original concept of Utility. Rule-Utilitarianism is also subject to the criticisms that face other rule based theories, such as that the rules may conflict (these will be discussed in more detail in the deontological ethics section). Attempts to provide a multi-level Utilitarianism with rule-Utility combined with a remainder rule allowing act-Utility to override rule-Utility in certain situations are too flexible and as such become little more than justification for intuitions.

4.2 Advantages and disadvantages of utilitarianism

Utilitarianism, as a monist theory with a single foundational principle, has the potential to provide the clinician with a simple and clear system with which to approach ethical dilemmas. This would allow the clinician to avoid the confusion of conflicting principles (in pluralistic theories such as Principalism). The Principle of Utility offers, in theory, to provide a reliable decision making procedure allowing the clinician to choose the correct course of action in every situation. Also Utility does not rely on a clinician's moral intuitions to identify or balance moral principles, which can sometime produce varying and unreliable outcomes. Utilitarianism is regarded as a very democratic system as each person's happiness has the same value; a King is not more valuable than a beggar. Utilitarianism shares, along with all Teleological Ethics, the valuable insight that the outcomes of our actions are important and should be taken into account in the ethical process.

As well as these considerable strengths, the greatest advantage of Utilitarianism is that it captures the heart of what ethics is for, being a system aiming to make people happy and alleviating suffering. These aims are in line with clinician's moral motivation to do good for patients and sum up for clinicians the purpose of medical ethics. Despite Teleological Ethic's rejection of the moral significance of motivation, Utilitarianism describes the strong desire to make people happy and reduce suffering that should be the starting point for a clinician's moral motivation.

Utilitarianism does, however, have a number of significant disadvantages and problems associated with it. The struggle to provide a coherent account of what is meant by happiness is an ongoing problem. It is by no means clear that happiness is the only good. Other goods, for example friendship or art, can be seen as goods in themselves, independent of the happiness they may or may not provide. In fact, it can be argued that it may be appropriate to suffer for such goods as friendship or art. There is also the issue of justification in Utilitarianism. For even if a satisfactory account of happiness as the good were provided, it would not necessarily follow that maximising happiness should be the overriding principle and so be considered morally obligatory.

However, a far greater problem for the clinician is that there is no way to measure happiness. There is no such thing as a Utility Calculator, and so with no units with which to measure happiness, so hedonistic calculus becomes meaningless in the clinical setting. Clinicians will also have the humility to realise that even the wisest person cannot know all the possible outcomes that will occur from an action. Evidence Based Medicine and Randomised Controlled Trials provide information with regards to the probabilities of a good clinical outcome from a medical intervention. However, applying such information to a patient cannot provide surety of happiness, as health is not the only good and the wider implications and long term outcomes often remain unknown. This is a problem with all Teleological Ethics. The future is essentially uncertain and so if all that matters about actions is their future consequences then morality is reduced to guesswork.

There are also significant problems with how happiness is distributed according to Utilitarian Calculus. Instead of "the greatest good for the greatest number", many situations arise in clinical practice in which the greatest good and the greatest number are in conflict. It is not clear whether total happiness or average happiness is the best and fairest outcome to strive for. According to simple hedonistic calculus the right action could often involve oppression of a minority for the benefit of a majority. According to Utilitarianism, Justice must be reduced to Utility, so violating the moral feelings of most clinicians and patients that equality and fairness are of great importance.

The principle of Utility followed through in clinical scenarios to its logical conclusions leads to a number of results that many clinicians find morally counter-intuitive. If consequences are all that matter, then for the sake of the best outcome many of the principles that govern human relationships, such as Justice or Rights, can be abandoned. In Utilitarianism, as in all Teleological Ethics, the ends always justify the means. This could lead to a clinician following hedonistic calculus to commit acts such as murder in the name of Utility, for example to provide organs to 5 other individuals. This would result in a loss of integrity that would be unacceptable to clinicians and to patients, the majority of whom would agree that this act is blatantly wrong.

Utilitarianism also has no mechanism for taking into account past actions in present decision making, as it is entirely focussed on future outcomes. This makes keeping a promise (such as maintaining the confidence of a patient), acting in gratitude or punishment difficult concepts to take account of in Utilitarianism, as they have no weight in hedonistic calculus. It is also possible that two acts that clinicians would consider opposite, for example attempting or not attempting Cardio-Pulmonary Resuscitation, can be given the same moral value according to hedonistic calculus, if their outcomes are the same (e.g. if the patient dies). Whilst Utilitarian's would argue that clinicians must let Utility challenge their common sense, if Utilitarianism demands such a complete rejection of the moral intuition of most clinicians and patients it loses any descriptive power to provide an account of moral feelings and intuitions.

Because Utilitarianism sees the happiness of all people as equal, there is no place in Utilitarianism for obligations arising from special relationships, e.g. to family, or to a patient. As well as this neglecting the doctor-patient relationship, it also creates a further problem that is compounded by the fact that in Utilitarianism there is no distinction between duty and supererogatory actions. This is the problem that Utilitarianism is too demanding, with too wide a scope, leaving clinicians morally responsible for all good outcomes that they were unable to achieve and for all negative outcomes that they failed to prevent. The scope of the demands of Utility cover anything that can suffer, so not just all people, but all animals create a demand to have their happiness maximised and their suffering relieved. Taken to its logical extremes the demands of Utility give no leave to a clinician to rest and no time for personal projects or the cultivation of special relationships (e.g. family and friends). Such a demand is not possible for a human to meet. However, it would be wrong to reject an ethical theory simply because it is not possible to measure up to its demands. Whilst in humility clinicians must remain aware of their finite resources and limitations, it is still beneficial to feel the demand of a Utilitarian Ethic that is both challenging and inspiring. An example of such a Utilitarian Ethic is Peter Singer's imperative for action to reduce third world poverty (Singer 1979).

4.3 Utilitarianism and QALYs

One of the areas in which Utilitarianism is considered the most useful is that of public policy and the distribution of resources. This is because it is a beneficence based theory, and when the goal is to produce as much good as possible with limited resources, Utilitarianism is by definition the best tool to use. Also in the sphere of public policy, where moral decisions are made abstracted from particular individuals and situations, many of the principles that govern human relationships, against which Utilitarianism seems to clash, are less apparent. However, Justice is key in such discussions and Utilitarian concepts of justice must continue to be weighed against other conceptions of justice.

QALYs (Quality Adjusted Life Years, as discussed earlier) are a cost-effectiveness analysis tool used in resource allocation and public policy decision making. QALYs are the best tool available to Utilitarianism to provide some measurement for Utilitarian Calculus. QALYs cannot be used in a strictly hedonistic Utilitarian Calculus, as they are not measures of pleasure. However, as a measure of years of life gained, weighted by the quality of the life gained, they are a powerful means of measuring and so weighing different consequences and as such provide a powerful tool to teleological ethics.

5. Deontological ethics

Deontological Ethics describes a group of ethical theories that judge actions as right or wrong on the basis of rules and duties. The word Deontology is derived from the Greek word *deon*, meaning duty. This means that, according to Deontology, it is not the outcomes of an action, but rather something intrinsic to the action itself, that makes it right or wrong. The intrinsic nature of the action is judged against a rule or set of rules, regardless of the outcome of that action. In order to act rightly, a moral agent must do their duty in accordance with the rules. The language of duty is used in some of the professional codes of conduct that govern clinicians' professional practice, for example in the UK the General Medical Council's "Duties of a Doctor." We will discuss deontological systems, starting with the most important, that of Immanuel Kant.

5.1 Kantian ethics (Kant 1785)

Kant argued that we can never know the full consequences of our actions and so, because we cannot know if our actions will have good or bad outcomes, we should perform actions that we know to be intrinsically good and avoid actions that we know to be intrinsically evil, and let the consequences unfold as they will. He argued that we know whether actions are good or bad from reason and not from their consequences. In fact, Kant based his ethical system entirely on reason. For Kant, reason was what defined a moral being and so he argued that reason underpinned the entire ethical endeavour and was sufficient for establishing moral law. He sought to use reason to work out a consistent, non-overridable set of moral rules that would be universal and binding to all rational creatures - a Supreme Moral Law. Kant argued that rational agents intrinsically possess absolute moral value and should recognise this in themselves and other rational agents. He argued then that the Supreme Moral Law should be obeyed out of duty alone, duty for duty's sake. For Kant it was not possible to be truly moral if acting out of self interest, or for any other motivation other than duty, even if the action is the same. The good will acts for the sake of the supreme moral law alone. Kant's Ethic can be described as "act as you wish, providing that your action conforms to the requirement of the Supreme moral law as represented by the categorical imperative" (Gillon 1985).

Kant's Ethical Theory is, therefore, an absolutist theory. Reason dictates the Supreme Moral Law, and this must be obeyed absolutely, out of duty alone. Kant's Theory is also a Monist Theory, a theory with only one principle. That principle is Kant's Categorical Imperative. Kant compares hypothetical imperatives, which indicate what ought to be done if a certain outcome is desired (if you want A, do B), with the categorical imperative, which is a simple binding command (do A) with no qualification. For Kant, hypothetical imperatives arise because we have desires for certain outcomes, but the categorical imperative arises from reason and as such is unqualified to demonstrate the weight of moral obligation. Kant, therefore, argued that this categorical imperative is absolute and immediate and all rational agents should understand it because of their rationality.

Kant has three formulations of his categorical imperative, which he saw as three ways of saying the same thing. The first of his formulations communicates the principle of universibility and is as follows, "act only according to the maxim by which you can at the same time will that it become a universal law". A maxim is a rule governing an individual's action and so a law is a maxim that passes the test of universibility. By this first formulation of the Categorical Imperative Kant argues that if rules are to have any validity and be considered as part of the Supreme Moral Law then they must be binding to all people at all times.

The second formulation of the Categorical Imperative expresses the value and dignity that Kant argued was intrinsic to rational agents. It is as follows, "So act as to treat humanity, whether in your own person or in that of any other, in every case as an end and never merely as a means". According to Kant human beings as rational agents embody the supreme moral law and have intrinsic moral worth, and so are the end that gives value to everything else, as means to the end of humanity. Humans, therefore, have unconditional worth, which is not derived from anybody or anything else's valuation of them.

The third formulation of the Categorical Imperative expresses Kant's Principle of Autonomy, "Every rational being is able to regard oneself as a maker of universal law". Kant's conception of autonomy is not simply the same as self-determination as discussed earlier in the section on Principalism. Rather he views only actions of moral self determination that are in line with reason as truly autonomous actions, expressing humanity's freedom as rational agents to act in accordance with duty to the Supreme Moral Law. Therefore, according to Kant, actions taken from passion, ambition or self interest all inhibit autonomous action. Kant sees the rational agent much like a King seeking to make laws for a Kingdom full of other rational agents.

When these three formulations of the Categorical Imperative are taken together Kant's rational agent must act like a King making rules to govern a Kingdom full of other rational agents, who will themselves be making rules in the same way. However, on the basis of the first formulation of universibility, Kant is confident that all the rules created by rational agents will not conflict, but rather be in harmony because all are derived from reason, which underpins the entire moral endeavour. This basis of reason for ethics means that Kant has no need for external authority for his ethics, such as the state, culture or God. God does, however, have a place in the Kantian system, even if He is not required as the basis of ethics. Kant requires God to bring justice by distribution of happiness to rational agents in accordance with their fulfilment of duty to the moral law (which doesn't happen in this life, but rather in the next).

5.2 Advantages and disadvantages of Kantian ethics

Kant's ethical theory provides an insight to clinicians that rules are important in ethics. Rules provide an excellent description of the expectations that most patients have of their doctors, e.g. don't break confidentiality, be honest. Reason provides Kant with a justification for many such moral rules, which in practice govern most human relationships, including the doctor-patient relationship. However, the greatest insights that Kantian ethics has to offer the clinician are demonstrated in the formulations of the categorical imperative. The first is that in order for an action to be judged right there must be good reason underlying it and this should be universible, so that a rule can be made that in a similar situation other people should act in the same way. This principle does not only apply when working within a Kantian System, and patients expect consistency from doctors dealing with similar cases. When such cases are compared doctors shave to be prepared to defend their decisions and the Bolam test defines the legal test that a reasonable body of other medical professionals would have acted in the same way. The second valuable insight of Kantian Ethics is Kant's Valuation of Humans as rational agents with absolute moral value. The insight of the second formulation of the categorical imperative, that people should never be treated merely as a means but rather as an end in themselves, has been a foundational principle in medical ethics and is in accord with the general feeling of clinicians with regards to the value of persons.

Kant's Ethical System can, however, be criticized for a number of reasons. That the Kantian system is far from clear limits its application to clinical practice. For example, the three formulations of the Categorical Imperative do not seem truly equivalent, as Kant argues and so the second and third formulations could be better thought of as supplementary principles that add content to Kant's morality. However the use of Kant's principles in this way brings in the problem of conflict between rules to the clinician. There are many clinical scenarios where obligation to one law derived from the categorical imperative, conflicts with an obligation to another law which is also derived from the categorical imperative, for example do not lie and do not break confidence. Kant's system provides no answer for this dilemma.

The first formalisation of the categorical imperative also seems to be too wide and too unqualified a principle upon which to develop of a moral law that could be applicable to clinical practice (Pojman 2006). It can be used to justify trivialities, even contradicting trivialities. Despite Kant's argument that consistency requires rules with no exceptions, there is nothing in the Categorical Imperative to prevent exceptions being added into maxims which still meet the requirements of Universalisation. However, this process is time consuming and impractical and of little benefit to the clinician facing an ethical dilemma.

As such Kant's system of derivation of rules from the categorical imperative is excessively formalistic, and thus lacks the implications on action necessary for appropriate application to the clinical setting. Kant's use of reason alone over-emphasises law and underemphasises relationships, as well as being unable to give an account of the moral importance of motivation. Most clinicians would regard a right action arising from sympathy, empathy and a desire to help their patient as more valuable that similar actions arising simply out of a sense of duty. Kant's focus on duty creates a version of morality that has been described as "austere and arid" (Gillon 1985), with no central place for beneficence or a desire to promote happiness or to love. This is perhaps the greatest criticism of Kant's ethical system for the clinician, namely that it seems to have missed the heart of moral motivation.

5.3 Some examples of other deontological systems

In contrast to Kant's Monist and Absolutist Theory, it is possible to create pluralist (with more than one rule) and objectivist (acknowledging that conflict between rules will occur) deontological theories. An example of such a theory is that of WD Ross. He distinguished between Prima Facie (at face value) and actual duties (Ross 1930). Prima Facie duties were derived from a number of rules/principles that it was the job of ethical discourse to elucidate. These duties were to be balanced against each other in specific situations to determine the actual/absolute duty in any given situation. The moral obligations listed by Ross include fidelity, beneficence, non-maleficence, justice (distribution of happiness in accord with merits/deserts), reparation, gratitude and self-improvement. Ross argued that these principles incorporate and reflect basic moral intuitions, but he denied that there is any overarching principle underlying them. He gave no account of how conflicts between principle are to be resolved except by citing the use of intuition, and he did not rank his principles in order of importance. The importance of Ross' Ethical System as an influence on the development of Principalism, demonstrates that Non-Absolutist Pluralist Deontological systems provide a useful platform for bridging with Utilitarianism and allowing the exploration of compatibility between these ethical systems in a clinical setting. Such exploration seems a promising avenue of inquiry for a clinician seeking for ethical resources when facing an ethical dilemma.

5.4 Rights theory

Rights Theory describes a set of claims that individuals (or groups) can make on other individuals (or groups). These claims are called rights. Rights Theory, often associated with the work of John Locke (Locke 1960) and his claims to life, liberty and estate, often seems to go hand in hand with liberal democracies and theories of liberal individualism. In such systems society's role is to provide space for individuals to pursue personal goods and projects. This space for the individual is protected by their rights.

There are different forms of rights. Legal rights can be enforced by law, but are created and abolished by the very parliaments, committees and dictators that write and enforce that law. Examples of legal rights are those enshrined in the Human Rights Act. Moral Rights (or natural rights) are rights that, it is argued, are possessed by everyone and cannot be taken away, even if they are ignored or trampled by governments or dictators.

Some Moral Rights are described as universal, meaning that they are attributable to all humans. An example of this is the right to autonomy (self-determination). However, there are also specific rights that are possessed by some and not others on the basis of special social relationships (e.g. the right of a child to be looked after by its parents/guardian or the doctor-patient relationship) or promises. The recipient of a promise has a right to claim what was promised, and legal promises (contracts) create legal rights which are enforceable by law. These specific rights are potentially universal, in the sense that anyone who receives such a promise or has such a special relationship will receive the same rights.

Some rights impose obligations on others to do something specific. These are called positive rights and they entitle the holder of such a right to receive a good or service from another. The other person is obliged to give the good or service demanded by the right. The specific rights based on a promise or a special relationship (e.g. the doctor-patient relationship) can be positive rights, but other rights which are claimed as universal, e.g. the right to healthcare or to education, also imply an obligation on someone else to provide this. However, it is not always clear who the other is that is obliged to provide the goods/services based on such universal positive rights.

Other rights require people not to do a certain thing. These are called Negative rights and they entitle the holder to be free from some action that others could potentially undertake.

The other person/people are obliged not to act in such a way. Examples of such rights are the right not to be killed or the right not to be tortured. Negative rights are in practice easier to enforce than positive rights. It is not always clear, however, whether rights are or should be positive or negative rights. For example, does John Locke's "life, liberty and estate" require other people not to kill, imprison or steal (negative rights) or does it require them to heal, liberate and provide (positive rights)?

Rights imply duties. Positive rights imply a duty on others to provide a good or service, and negative rights create a duty on other not to act in a certain way. Rights theory has been included in the section on deontological ethics for this reason. It is not clear whether rights could provide the basis for the rules which underpin deontological theories, or whether rights arise from such rules. However, clinicians need to be aware that a relationship between rights and duties does exist, because when a patient claims a right to healthcare, the duty will fall to the clinician to provide.

Often rights are claimed as absolutes and so any action against rights is seen as a direct violation of the right itself. This allows rights to be used as a trump card against society, protecting the individual. However, this creates problems for the clinician because in many clinical situations the rights of one individual impinge on the rights of another, just as in deontological theories rules can often conflict with each other. An example of this could be the right of a patient diagnosed with an STI to confidentiality and the right of their partner to know of the risk to their health. Rights may be seen by the clinician, however, as valuable but not absolute principles, which often have to be weighed against each other, much in the same way as Ross' Prima Facie Duties. So certain rights may on occasion need to be impinged, especially when they conflict, but this must always be justified and rights remain as a constant reminder to the clinician of the dignity and equality due to all individuals.

5.5 Advantages and disadvantages of rights theory

The great strength of right's theory is the protection for individuals that it provides, especially in the light of the great abuses that have been done to individuals throughout history in the name of the "greater good", by society or even by the medical profession (e.g. in Nazi Germany). Rights represent the promise from the majority to the minority, from the powerful to the weak, that their dignity and equality will be respected. Since doctors are often in positions of significant power over patients, the rights of the patient are an important reminder of the duty and respect due to the patient that the doctor's power implies. Rights have often encouraged the oppressed and maltreated to stand up and protest, which serves and important and beneficial role in a society, although this can be uncomfortable for the powerful members of that society.

However, Rights Theory cannot provide clinicians with a complete ethical theory in itself. It provides no account of the role of emotion, supererogatory action or virtue, instead providing only minimally enforceable rules. In its protection of the individual it excludes and ignores group interests and communal values. By focussing on what an individual is owed, it changed the focus of morality from one of duty, responsibility and a desire to do good, into an egotistical focus on what can be demanded. Rights could, therefore, be one factor underlying an increasingly consumer based culture driving healthcare in the developed world. Whilst protecting the value of patients , Right Theory cannot account for or exhort clinicians to the beneficent drive to strive of the best for their patients, which is the heart of moral motivation.

In this way right's theory can be best seen by the clinician as an outworking of one of the great insights of deontological ethics, that of human value. Right's Theory puts flesh on the bones of how this principle is worked out in human society, where valuable humans live side by side. Rights theory dictates the boundaries of protection for individuals from others, limiting what can be done to them in the name of a "greater good", and negative rights are a valuable tool in this. Positive rights, however, especially when taken out of the sphere of specific rights into universal rights, have difficulty identifying who has the duty to fulfil the right. In a resource limited world many of the universal positive rights that are claimed are often seen as aspirational rather than realistic. Therefore, a universal positive right implies a duty (perhaps on all) to try to provide the good demanded, but because of the scale and practical impossibilities, of for example providing healthcare to all, does not create a duty on clinicians to actually provide all people with the services required. Rights can provide a coherent imperative to the clinician against doing wrong to a patient, but often fail to provide a coherent imperative to exhort good to be done to that patient.

5.6 How the clinician could use utilitarianism and deontological ethics

Whilst Utilitarianism and Deontological Ethics seem so divergent as to be almost opposites, they both highlight different insights of Ethical Theory which are of great importance to the clinician in medical ethics. Utilitarianism, with its emphasis on the importance of outcomes and its focus on maximising happiness and relieving suffering, expresses the heart of moral motivation and embodies much of the beneficent drive that motivates clinicians to seek the best outcomes for their patients. Utilitarianism also has special use in the particular area of the development of public policy and resource allocation.

Deontological Ethics, in particular Kantian Ethics, claims that ethical decisions should be justifiable by reason and, therefore, be universal. Deontology gives expression to many of the rules that in practice govern human relationships and describe well the expectations of patients and clinicians of the doctor-patient relationship. The most importance insight of deontology is the value of humans. From this can be derived the importance of non-maleficence, respect for autonomy and justice. In this way Deontological Ethics act as a check on the beneficent drive and moral motivation to do good, in terms of creating happiness and relieving suffering, that arises from Utilitarianism, preventing it from reaching counterintuitive conclusions or disregarding the value of human beings. Utilitarianism describes the starting moral motivation of the clinician, but deontological ethics ensures that this is worked out in the right way. This can perhaps be expressed by adapting Gillon's Summary of the Kantian Ethic "Act as you wish providing that your action conforms to the requirements of the moral law" to include a Utilitarian motivation. This could be expressed as "A clinician should act to maximise happiness and relieve suffering providing that such action conforms to the requirements of the value of humanity of the patient, in terms of duties to the principles of Non-Maleficence, respect for Autonomy and Justice".

This is similar to the earlier proposal that, in Principalism, Beneficence forms the starting point and motivation in an ethical dilemma but must be weighed against the other principles of Non-Maleficence, Autonomy and Justice in order to ensure that the ethical weight of these perspectives is not overlooked. Whilst not providing a defining solution to dilemmas in medical ethics, and seemingly leaving the clinician weighing between principles as does Principalism, discussing and seeking to balance Utilitarianism and

Deontology provides additional depth to the clinician's understanding of the Four Principles. Seeing Beneficence in terms of maximising happiness and relieving suffering and seeing Non-Maleficence, Autonomy and Justice in terms of valuing humanity allows the clinician to have a better understanding of what the Four Principles are for and so when choosing one principle over another may be appropriate. In some situations the imperative to maximise happiness and relieve suffering will be so powerful that it should not be tempered, but in other situations overriding Non-Maleficence or respect for Autonomy would devalue the humanity of a patient in an unacceptable manner.

This still, however, leaves clinicians weighing between principles. In order to provide further resources to such a clinician a change in perspective is necessary. Such a change in perspective is provided by Virtue Ethics.

6. Virtue ethics

Virtue Ethics is a description of a way of thinking ethically that, rather than focussing on the rules or outcomes relating to specific actions, focuses on character and motivation. Actions are judged in the light of character, meaning that the right action in a situation is defined as the action that, in that situation, a virtuous person would take. A virtuous person is described according to the Virtues (good character traits or moral habits, for example kindness, generosity, courage, justice, prudence, etc), and it is from these virtues that Virtue Ethics takes its name.

According to Virtue Ethics it is not just important to do the right thing, but to have the right disposition, motivation and emotions to be a good person who does the right thing. This makes Virtue Ethics well suited to both Public and Private Life, bridging the gap between the two and demanding integrity in both. Virtues such as justice and beneficence define the virtuous person's public life, whilst the virtues of love and care direct their private lives. Virtue Ethics is an ethics of aspiration, not an ethic of duty. In order to become a virtuous person it is necessary to discover a proper moral example and imitate that. Becoming a virtuous person involves an apprentice-like training in virtue. Imitating the right model results in a virtuous person, who has trained to spontaneously do good.

Virtue Ethics was brought to prominence in modern ethics by Elizabeth Anscombe and Alasdair MacIntyre. They argued that since the enlightenment moral philosophy had become unable to provide a meaningful moral imperative, and that a return to virtue ethics was the only possible way forward (MacIntyre 2011). Virtue Ethics, as an inspiring ethical theory that took ethics away from legal context and embraced both the importance of spirituality as well as the value of community, was therefore, proposed as an alternative to the flawed deontic (action based) systems.

The modern resurgence of Virtue Ethics, relies on theories of Virtue Ethics that date back to Ancient Greece. Both Plato and Aristotle discussed the virtues, but it is Aristotle who is considered the father of Virtue Ethics.

6.1 Aristotelian ethics (Aristotle 1998)

The concept of a *telos* (goal or end) underpins all of Aristotle's ethics. The *telos* in Aristotle's ethics is different, however, from the use that is made of the word telos in teleological ethics, where *telos* describe the focus on the goals or outcome of actions. The *telos* for Aristotle describes the goal towards which all of humanity is moving. It is this goal that gives the meaning and purpose to humans that is necessary to provide the ethical imperative to be a virtuous person. The *telos* towards which Aristotle describes all humanity moving, he calls *Eudaimonia*. *Eudaimonia* means literally having a good angel, but describes a state of human flourishing, happiness, well-being and blessedness – the good life. For Aristotle, therefore, humanity has an essence or a function, to pursue *eudaimonia*, the good life. This human flourishing is a much richer concept than the simple happiness described by Utilitarianism. It describes health, wealth, social well-being and growth in virtue. Aristotle's conception of human flourishing, however, is coloured by his context of life in an Athenian City State and can seem egotistical in focus. It is possible, however, for the concept of human flourishing to be developed beyond this and for the virtuous person to be governed by a *telos* that desires and seeks flourishing in all of these ways not just for the self, but for others around, and for all of humanity.

For Aristotle, in order to lead a human life well, and so to pursue *eudaimonia*, the virtues are necessary. He describes the good of man (humanity) as "the activity of the soul in conformity with virtue". Aristotle defines the virtues as a trait of character manifested in habitual action, that it is good for a person to have. These virtues are the qualities needed for successful human living, and Aristotle describes the virtues as the good mean between two negative vices, represented by deficiency and excess. For example, courage is the mean between cowardice and foolhardiness. Other virtues that Aristotle describes include generosity, honesty, self control and loyalty to friends or family. Friendship is of great importance to Aristotle, and he argues that no-one would choose to live without friends, even if he had all other goods.

Aristotle acknowledges that we do not have direct control over our emotions, and are susceptible to temptation with dispositions that cannot be simply turned on or off. However, he argues that we do have indirect control over our emotions, and it is possible to take steps to develop the right dispositions and attitudes, as well as correcting wrong ones. This can be a long and difficult process that Aristotle describes by the metaphor of a garden. The emotions are plants that grow of their own accord. They will grow wild if left alone, but the virtuous person is the gardener who works to guide and control the plants, cutting some back and encouraging others to grow more. Such an account of emotion and its role in the ethical life is missing in deontic systems and is a powerful description of the importance and role of emotion in ethical development. A further ethical imperative is discovered by Virtue Ethics here. We must not simply do the good, nor is being good sufficient, we must learn to love the good.

Aristotle grounds his concept of the quest for the good life and growth in the virtues in real life. The virtuous person, whilst always focussed on the *telos* of human flourishing, is constantly engaged in real life situations and circumstances. *Phronesis* (practical wisdom) is how Aristotle describes the virtuous person's ability to respond realistically to specific circumstances, whilst remaining directed and guided by the *telos* of human flourishing. *Phronesis* allows the virtuous person to find the right means with which to accomplish the right ends, as demanded by the virtues (Kaldijan 2010).

6.2 Advantages and disadvantages of virtue ethics

As discussed earlier, Virtue Ethics has the great advantage for the clinician of providing an account of the importance of moral motivation to the ethical life. It values friendship, love, respect and mutual regard in relationships and values action taken for those reasons, rather than just from a sense of duty. Virtue Ethics also points to the importance of moral saints and heroes as inspiring examples for clinicians to imitate. One such moral example for clinicians is set by the life of Albert Schweitzer, who as a doctor, philosopher and theologian spent many years in Africa working to help the impoverished there. His life not only provides an informative example of a virtuous person, but one that inspires clinicians to imitate it. In doing this, Virtue Ethics creates an emphasis on the importance of moral development that is missing in deontic ethics.

Virtue Ethics also provides the clinician with a different perspective by addressing some of the weaknesses of deontic ethics, including broadening the scope of ethics from a now defunct "legal" context borrowed from theology, over-emphasising autonomy and neglecting communal goods (as described above). Virtue Ethics also provides a good account of and potential solution to the tension in many deontic systems between partiality and impartiality. Utilitarianism in particular has no place for special relationships such as the doctor-patient relationship, or special duties arising from such a relationship. This seems to miss something important about the importance of the doctor-patient relationship, and Virtue Ethics can both fill in the gap and explain the tension. Different virtues can be used to both emphasise the importance of impartiality (such as beneficence and justice), whilst others demonstrate the importance of partiality (including love and friendship). The virtuous clinician will exhibit all these virtues and by *phronesis* work out when it is right to be impartial (for example in public policy making) and when it is right to fulfil duties based on special relationships (for example in the doctor-patient relationship).

Criticisms of Virtue Ethics are that it cannot give a complete account of the ethical life for a clinician. In particular it cannot provide a complete account of the importance of doing the right thing and the place of rules in ethical decision making. The focus of Virtue Ethics is away from the moment of decision about whether a particular action is right or wrong. Thus turning to Virtue Ethics for guidance in that moment can often yield little guidance to the clinician. The answer to "do what a virtuous person would do", can be of very little help, when it is unclear what a virtuous person would do, or when two virtuous clinician differ in opinion about what should be done.

Virtue Ethics also contains a number of different virtues. Whilst this adds richness and explanatory power to describe a number of tensions within human experience, relationships and the ethical life, it can also creates uncertainty about what to do when virtues clash. This is a similar problem to that faced by pluralist deontological theories and right's theories, as a weighing between the claims of different virtues is required in order to decide the right course of action, and no clear account of how this is to be done is given. Aristotle's concept of *phronesis* foresees this problem and provides a concept with which the clinician can be equipped when facing dilemmas between virtues in specific circumstances. The concept of *phronesis* is not, however, fleshed out to the degree whereby it could provide a clear process for such decision making. Rather it is more of an acknowledgement that a virtuous clinician, when seeking the *telos* of human flourishing and exhibiting the virtues, should be trusted to face and overcome such dilemmas.

6.3 How the clinician could use virtue ethics to complement deontic ethics

In order to overcome the apparent incompleteness of a solitary account of either deontic or Virtue Ethics, attempts have been made to combine the two. Differing weight can be given to either deontic or virtue ethics in such a combination, and this gives rise to theories with different emphases. Correspondence Theories describe a combination of virtue and deontic ethics where deontic, in particular deontological emphasis on rules or principles, is given precedence over Virtue Ethics. The virtues, therefore, are seen as habits of obedience to certain principles or rules, and as such the virtues are derived from those rules or principles. Virtues have a motivational role, which could otherwise be lacking in a purely deontological theory, as they inspire people to obey the rules. Possessing the virtues makes a person more likely to obey the rules and in doing so the virtues have value in Correspondence Theories.

Complementary or Pluralistic Ethical Theories describe theories in which the virtues have an equal role alongside rules or principles, as necessary in order to live the good life. The virtues are not simply derivative or instrumental, but describe duties to be certain kinds of people that are equally as important as duties to behave in certain kinds of ways. Such a Complementary Theory could place the virtues alongside the principles arising in a pluralist non-absolutist deontological theory, giving rise to the prima facie duties that must be weighed in order to determine the actual/absolute duty in any given situation. As such Virtue Ethics can perhaps best be seen as part of an overall theory of ethics rather than a complete theory in itself. Virtue Theory, therefore, would find its place in ethical theory alongside an adequate conception of right action arising from Deontic Ethics.

Just as Utilitarianism can be seen to provide the clinician with an explanation of the ethical drive to do good, and Deontological Ethics provides guidance in how that good is to be worked out in light of the value of persons, justice, and the importance of universibility in ethical decisions, Virtue Ethics also provides important additional resources to the clinician. The development of character and growth in the virtues by imitation of a virtuous role model describes very well the apprentice-like way that much of clinical practice is learned by junior and student clinicians. Aristotle's description of the good life as the pursuit of excellence in accordance with the virtues, describes well the twin needs of clinical trainees to develop both in clinical skill as well as in character and moral habit. By introducing this perspective into the framework already provided by Utilitarian and Deontological Ethics, Virtue Ethics broadens the clinician's view of the role and importance of ethics. The relevance of ethics is no longer limited to problematic situations, but should also govern the entire life of the clinician, encouraging development of character and moral habit to allow a clinician to become a virtuous clinician. Virtue Ethics provides the motivation, inspiration and an account of the role of emotions that are all necessary for such character development.

Virtue Ethics adds something of greater importance to Utilitarianism and Deontological ethics. Virtue Ethics adds the perspective of a *telos*, a goal or purpose, for humanity, that of human flourishing. This *telos* is a guide in ethical decision making and by *phronesis* the virtuous person engages with the realities of the situation they are faced with, while still striving to act to bring about human flourishing. This provides a model for clinicians when faced with ethical dilemmas and the balancing of different principles. A decision should be made, guided by the *telos* of human flourishing, using practical reasoning (*phronesis*) which is a learned ability that clinicians develop. This model emphasises the importance of character development and growth in virtue and moral habits and these produce not only the development of *phronesis*, but also transform clinicians into virtuous people, who are the ones who should be trusted to make such ethical decisions. As clinicians we should strive to make ethical decisions, guided by the *telos* of human flourishing. We should make our aim to make ethical decisions that help our patients to flourish in health, happiness and also in moral development. It is as we do this that we will also flourish into virtuous clinicians.

7. Conclusion

This chapter has discussed a number of ethical resources that are available to clinicians. These resources have relevance to all clinicians from students encountering some of the medical ethics dilemmas for the first time to experienced clinicians striving for the good of their patients. Each theory has its own merits, but also its own limitations, and no theory alone is able to provide all the answers necessary when striving for the good in clinical practice. However, in trying to hold some of the theories together a clinician can gain from the cumulative strength of a number of theories, and so find a balanced perspective, free from the weaknesses of individual theories.

This chapter discussed the Four Principles: Beneficence, Non-maleficence, Justice and Autonomy , which provide a useful analytical tool in ethical dilemmas. These principles are useful to the clinician in that they draw from a number of ethical theories. However, they leave the clinician with a dilemma in how the principles are to be balanced when they come into conflict. This problem arises from Ross' system of Prima Facie duties, on which Principalism is heavily dependent. The chapter also discussed Values-Based Medicine which is a useful outworking of what the Principle of Autonomy looks like in clinical practice and patient interactions.

Utilitarianism was also explored, with its fundamental principle of utility, seeking to maximise happiness and relieve suffering. This principle captures the heart of moral motivation in the desire to act ethically. The outworkings of this principle of utility, when given free reign in ethical thinking, may lead to many counterintuitive results, and this is why comparison and combination with Deontological Ethics adds balance to Utilitarianism. Kant's Deontological system, in particular, provides important insights into the value of persons, the importance of justice, and the need for ethical decisions to pass the test of universibility. Rights Theory is important as a further outworking of this insight into the value of humans, and seeks to prevent abuse of the individual for the "greater good" of society. Using these insights as principles in a non-absolute, pluralist deontological system (such as that described by Ross) allows them to balance and temper the clinicians desire to do good (as encapsulated by utilitarianism). This creates a system that is not dissimilar to the Four Principles of Beauchamp and Childress balanced by Gillon's method, using Beneficence/Utility as the driving motivation of the clinician, tempered by Non-Maleficence, Justice and Autonomy (which arise from deontological ethics).

Virtue Ethics opens up a different perspective in ethical discussion to cover not just the process of making an ethical decision, but also to cover character development and growth in virtue through the whole life of the clinician. In doing so, Virtue Ethics points clinicians not just to the virtues as abstract principles, but also as displayed in the lives of virtuous senior clinicians from whom the virtues can be learnt by imitation as apprentices. The examples of moral saints and heroes are part of the inspiration and motivation that virtue ethics adds to the potentially negative and uninspiring discussion of the action-based deontological and utilitarian systems. Virtue Ethics also provides a model with which to approach ethical dilemmas that arise from situations where principles conflict and must be weighed against each other. The virtuous clinician must use their practical wisdom (*phronesis*) to assess the realities of the situation in the light of the goal or essence (*telos*) of humanity, which is human flourishing. Virtue Ethics places trust in the virtuous clinician, who has worked hard to develop these virtues and to grow in the practical wisdom necessary to decide how to maximise human flourishing and in particular the flourishing of their patients.

8. Acknowledgement

I am grateful to Dr Fistein for her ongoing help and support.

9. References

Aristotle (1998). Nichomachean Ethics, Dover Thrift Editions, ISBN 0-486-40096-4, USA

Beauchamp, T., & Childress J. (2009). Principles of Biomedical Ethics (Sixth Edition), Oxford University Press ISBN-13:978-0-19-533570-5, New York

Bentham, J. (1789). An Introduction to the Principles of Morals and Legislation, Bottom of the Hill Publishing, ISBN: 978-1-61203-030-2, USA

De Grazia D. (2003). Common Morality, coherence and the principles of biomedical ethics. Kennedy Inst Ethics J, 13:219e30

Donaldson, T., Fistein E., & Dunn, M. (2010). Case-based seminars in medical ethics education: how medical students define and discuss moral problems. J Med Ethics, 36:816-820 originally published online October 20,2010 doi: 10.1136/jme.2010.036574

Fulford, K., (2004). FACTS/VALUES Ten Principles of Values-Based Medicine, In: The Philosophy of Psychiatry, Radden J., pp. (205-234), Oxford University Press, ISBN No. 0-19-514953-x

Gillon, R. (1985). Philosophical Medical Ethics, John Wiley and Sons ISBN 0 471 91222 0, Great Britain

Kaldijan L.C. (2010). Teaching practical wisdom in medicine through clinical judgement, goals of care, and ethical reasoning. J Med Ethics, 36:558-562

Kant, I. (1795) Groundwork of the Metaphysics of Moral, Cambridge University Press ISBN 0 521 62695 1, UK

Kant I (1788). Critique of Practical Reason, Cambridge University Press ISBN 0 521 59051 5, UK

Locke J (1960). Two Treatises of Government, Cambridge University Press ISBN 978-0-521-35730-2, USA

MacIntyre, A. (2011). After Virtue (Third Edition), Bloomsbury ISBN 978 0 7156 3640 4, Great Britain

Mill, JS. (1861). Utilitarianism, Hackett Publishing Company, Inc, ISBN-13:978-0-87220-695-2, Indianapolis

Pojman, LP. (2006). Ethics Discovering Right and Wrong (Fifth Edition), Thomson Wadsworth ISBN 0-534-61936-3, USA

Rachels, J. (2003). The Elements of Moral Philosophy (Fourth Edition), McGraw-Hill Higher Education ISBN 0-07-247690-7, New York

Ross, W. D. (1930). The Right and the Good, Oxford University Press, London

Singer P. (1979). Practical Ethics, Cambridge University Press ISBN 0 521 29720 6, USA

3

Neuroenhancement – A Controversial Topic in Contemporary Medical Ethics

Kirsten Brukamp and Dominik Gross
Institute for History, Theory, and Ethics of Medicine,
RWTH Aachen University,
Germany

1. Introduction

Neuroenhancement will become an important topic of medical ethics in future years and decades, due to the increasing insights of neuroscience into the functions of the brain and the growing possibilities of meaningful interventions. Consequently, several crucial topics need to be discussed in order to address this emerging issue, and these topics correspond to the following sections of this article:

1. Introduction
2. Enhancement: How is enhancement defined? Which topics in the theory of medicine does it touch on, and which concepts help to understand it better?
3. Neuroenhancement and its categories: What is neuroenhancement in particular? What are the ends and methods of neuroenhancement? Which subtypes exist, and how can they be classified?
4. Pharmacological and technological neuroenhancement: Which medication is used for pharmacological neuroenhancement? How may technological advancements be utilized to achieve neuroenhancement?
5. Principles in medical ethics: How are ethical judgments usually made in medical ethics? According to which criteria should neuroenhancement be assessed in general?
6. Ethical assessment of neuroenhancement: Which arguments are used to support or criticize neuroenhancement? What are the advantages and disadvantages? How can neuroenhancement currently be assessed and judged?
7. Conclusion

2. Enhancement

Enhancement strategies in medicine, in general, are opposed to the classic framework of medical interventions - namely therapeutic, preventive, rehabilitative, and palliative measures –, in so far as no medical reasons, i.e. indications, for them exist: The people who request enhancements are not affected by disease according to classic standards and have not received a medical diagnosis related to their wishes. The intention behind enhancements is the improvement of subjective well-being and a higher quality of life. Although a general definition differentiates between therapy and enhancement, the dividing line needs to be outlined separately for each type of treatment. A "treatment" for enhancement purposes is not synonymous with "therapy" any longer. Examples for enhancement include aesthetic surgery, doping in sports, and the use of presumed anti-aging medication.

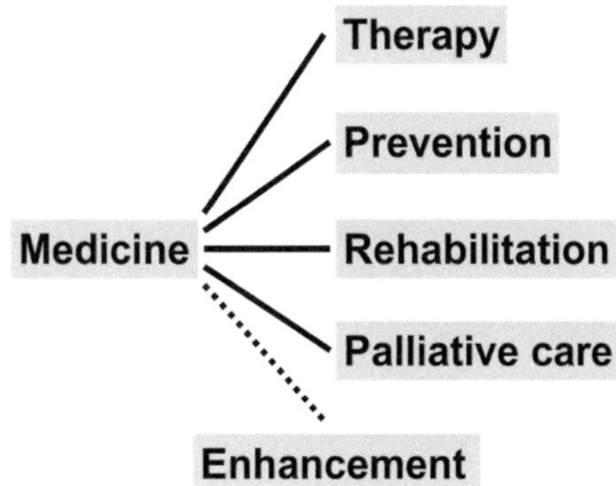

Fig. 1. Medicine comprises a multitude of different concepts for the wide notion of health care. Enhancement, however, is not usually considered a classic part of this, even though overlaps exist in expertise and methods.

The "enhancement" concept elicits a number of questions in the realm of the theory of medicine (Groß, 2011): What is a "disease" state, as opposed to "health"? Can a state of "normalcy" be defined? Are these views not culture-sensitive and changing throughout history? In addition, social and ethical concerns follow: In which way is the physician-patient relationship going to change when more enhancement options become available? Is the "patient" concept in medicine replaced by a "client" concept?

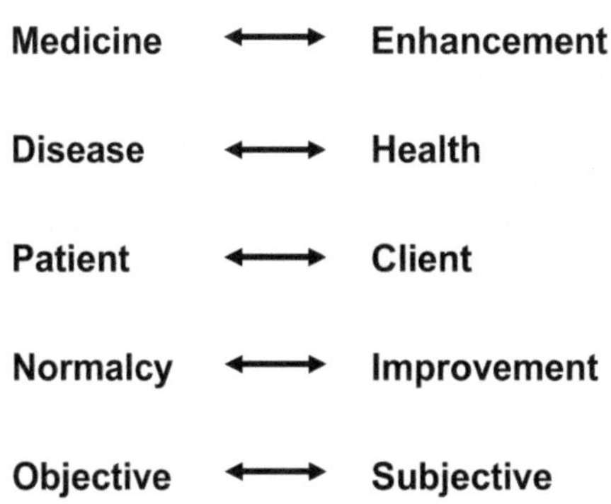

Fig. 2. The difference between medicine and enhancement may, in simplified form, be portrayed by antonyms, although the conceptual distinction is complex and possesses many implications, which still need to be pondered in the theory of medicine.

Distinguishing between therapy and enhancement is culture-dependent. The differences between them cannot be determined by science alone. Rather, it is the role of science to provide data about biological and medical facts. Based on this, societies then decide which functional states count as "normal", "variant", "different", or "diseased", just to name a few possibilities for overall assessments. These judgments are difficult to make, given the complexities that result from an interaction between phenotypical features that are problematic to classify individually themselves. Three specific examples deserve mention: complications of features, population biology, and life stages.

Complications of features: A population may possess a feature M in the majority of cases, with a complication rate of X% for a serious health problem, which is undesirable according to public opinion. In addition, there may be a variant feature V in a minority, with a higher complication rate of (X+Y)% for the serious complication. How is social acceptance for feature V achieved on the individual or the population level? When does feature V become a disease? Does this depend on the percentage with which it occurs in the population, on the seriousness of the complication, or on the complication rate? These questions cannot be contemplated within science alone; the answers require a qualified insight into the practices, needs, and desires of a culture.

Population biology: From a population standpoint, e.g. in evolution, it is advantageous to produce a variability of features, within certain limits. This makes the population more stable in its niche. The features that are currently present have developed over many generations and are balanced with each other. Under these circumstances, simultaneous, congruent shifts in features can reduce adaptive capacities and may be detrimental for a population as a whole, although they could certainly be beneficial at times as well. When are such feature shifts healthy or abnormal? - In parallel, it is unclear what the sequelae will be when a significant number of humans want to change their appearances, skills, or habits in a certain direction at the same time through enhancement. From a societal perspective, it may be better to discourage such a desire.

Life stages: It remains unclear how to classify changes that occur relatively often during temporary stages of life only, for example childhood and puberty, pregnancy and old age. Is lower extremity edema during pregnancy normal or a disease? Is cognitive decline with increasing age normal, or is old age a disease with dementia as one of its signs? These puzzles illustrate that the dividing line between health and disease becomes blurry in special, but still fairly common situations. Sometimes, it is best to explain states in terms of their physiology and pathophysiology rather than to apply a biased term too early.

In summary, the concept of enhancement is vague because the notion of disease in medicine is debated as well. In addition, the intentions for enhancements are subjective: What counts as an improvement for one person may be unacceptable for another.

3. Neuroenhancement and its categories

Neuroenhancement is the use of enhancement strategies - according to the definition for enhancement in general - that affect the nervous system. More specifically, such a use, in the narrow sense, mostly concerns the central nervous system because there are limited potential applications in the peripheral nervous system. Classifications of neuroenhancement may be developed according to two distinct categories: 1. the cognitive functions that are to be improved as well as the intentions and aims that underlie the use and 2. the methods or routes that are employed. The different methods may result in permanent or temporary enhancement.

Categories of neuroenhancement according to cognitive functions

1. Sensory perception
2. Motor action
3. Communication
4. Mood and emotions
5. Cognition, narrowly conceived (e.g. attention, memory, decision-making)
6. Social and moral behavior

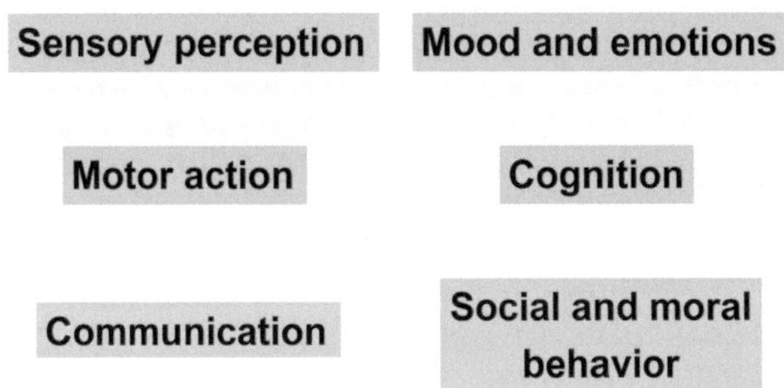

Fig. 3. Categories of neuroenhancement according to cognitive functions.

This classification by cognitive roles and intentions covers all major functions that the central nervous system usually exercises. One overarching aim is to improve the interaction between the subject and the environment: A human needs to communicate effectively with her surroundings; both sensory uptake and motor output help this purpose. The other central aim is to expand the overall behavioral repertoire. This allows the person to act more freely and gives her more options to choose from - cognitively, socially, and morally.

Neuroenhancement regarding *sensory perception* may mean to improve the functioning of the human senses or to potentially acquire new types of perception. For example, visual and auditory senses could be enhanced to include new wavelengths and frequencies outside the usual visible and audible spectrum. Regarding olfaction, humans may imitate dogs; as with all types of enhancement, however, it needs to be seen why they would want to procure this particular ability. - *Motor neuroenhancement* could lead to more efficient steering of technical devices. This type of use is largely futuristic; nevertheless, medical reports on tetraplegia (Hochberg et al., 2006) demonstrate that brain-machine interfaces can be utilized as therapies in order to expand the motor skills of severely compromised, wheelchair-bound patients. - *Communication*, enhanced by neurotechnology, appears as a promise with a high commercial potential. After all, recent years have seen a rise in communication technology, both towards large social networks and in favor of brief messages of an informational or emotional nature. Both trends could potentially continue with neuroenhancement.

Emotions and mood are typically improved for therapeutic purposes in depressive patients. The slogan "Feeling 'better than well'" (Hall, 2004) seems to suggest that people who consider their emotions as normal may feel even happier, more euphoric, or generally enhanced when they take antidepressants. - *Cognitive functions* in the narrow sense, such as attention and memory, may become better through neuroenhancement as well. Some pharmaceutical drugs developed for medical purposes do improve concentration, at least temporarily (Repantis et al., 2010). Medication that reduces the need for sleep also belongs to this general category. So-called "memory chips" are still very much a matter of speculation: These devices would store information outside of the brain, and they would allow access to deposit and retrieve these data (Groß, 2009b). - Social neuroscience aims at elucidating the determinants of living in groups and cultures. Eventually, the scientific results could be translated into opening up options for favorable *social and moral behavior*.

A further classification of neuroenhancement relies on the methods that proponents pursue to achieve the goal.

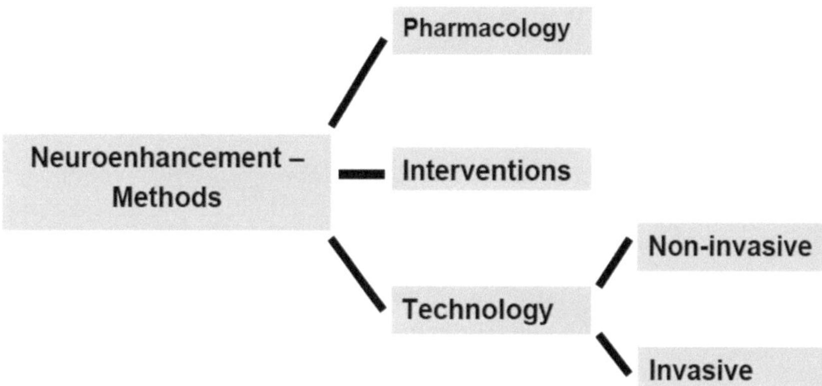

Fig. 4. Categories of neuroenhancement according to the methods employed.

Categories of neuroenhancement according to the methods employed

1. Pharmacology
2. Interventions (surgical or minimally invasive)
3. Non-invasive, external technology
4. Invasive, internal technology

In the following, the focus will be on pharmacological measures and implanted technology.

4. Pharmacological and technological neuroenhancement

Pharmacological neuroenhancement is known under different names, such as "cosmetic neurology" and "brain doping". These latter terms clearly reflect the enhancement character of the endeavor. The medications used belong to a variety of medical classes, including pharmaceutical drugs used against depression (e.g. fluoxetine), dementia (e.g. donepezil), attention-deficit hyperactivity disorder (e.g. methylphenidate), and narcolepsy and sleeping disorders (e.g. modafinil) (Groß, 2009a).

Neuroenhancing medication, therefore, is already a reality to a degree - as evidenced by the prevalence for the use of methylphenidate, modafinil, and antidepressants for this purpose particularly in the United States of America (Greely et al., 2008). The drugs are used in schools, at universities, and at work for similar purposes: to improve objective performance parameters and to boost self-esteem.

Interventions for neuroenhancement may be performed by microsurgery; however, these techniques do not yet exist. *Non-invasive, external technology* comprises brain stimulation techniques, such as transcranial magnetic stimulation (TMS) and transcranial direct current stimulation (tDCS). Although these methods possess potential to enhance brain function, they have not been developed to a degree to allow a reliable use for enhancement at the present time.

The *technological* advancements that support neuroenhancement are largely futuristic. As discussed above, they can be categorized into attempts to improve sensory, motor, communicative, emotional, cognitive, and social functions. The technological products that are already available suggest that some enhancement strategies may be successful more readily than others. In particular, the following applications come to mind: supersensory perception, prosthesis steering, and more efficient communication.

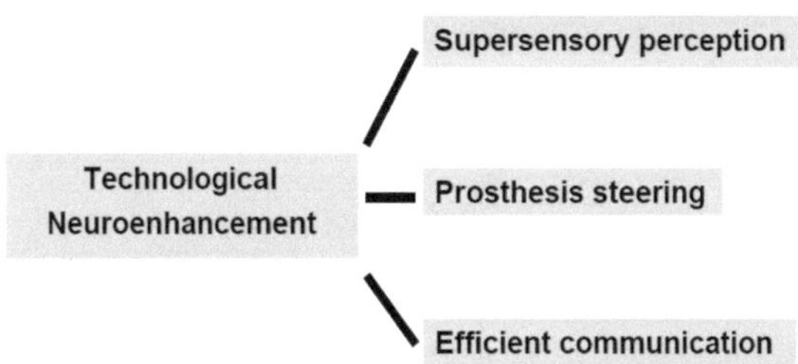

Fig. 5. Pursuits in technological neuroenhancement that are currently in development.

Supersensory perception is already on the horizon, given the medical treatments of retinal, cochlear, and auditory brainstem implants (Groß, 2007a). Both humans (Hochberg et al., 2006) and non-human primates (Velliste et al., 2008) have been capable of using brain-machine interfaces to *steer prosthesis*. Brain signals can be analyzed for motor-independent *communication* (Monti et al., 2010).

Emotions and mood may be changed by internal devices as well. In curative medicine, deep brain stimulation is an accepted treatment for Parkinson's disease and essential tremor as well as other diseases (Deep-Brain Stimulation for Parkinson's Disease Study Group, 2001). Deep brain stimulation is administered through electrodes that are implanted in deep regions of the brain, such as basal ganglia. Its effects include neurological and psychological ones, such as both positive and negative influences as well as side effects on extrapyramidal motor functions and emotional activation, which oftentimes manifests as euphoria and mania (Müller & Christen, 2011). Accordingly, a mild mode of stimulation might improve mood without other detrimental side effects. At this time, however, a wide-spread use of rather large, invasive electrodes is not conceivable for enhancement purposes. Regarding *cognitive functions*, memory chips have been discussed, but continue to remain elusive for now. *Social and moral behavior* is so complex and adaptable that it is currently unclear how to specifically enhance it, outside of general effects on emotional and cognitive states.

Neurotechnology has already been demonstrated to exhibit rather upsetting effects in some cases. In rats, a selective microstimulation technology for select brain areas has been used to coerce the animals into following certain paths that they would otherwise have shied away from (Talwar et al., 2006). Such applications lead to criticism against brain interventions *per se.*

5. Principles in medical ethics

Neuroenhancement can be assessed according to standard approaches in medical ethics, e.g. principlism, a strong contemporary attitude in medical ethics. It takes into consideration four principles, which draw widespread approval even from divergent ideological positions, namely autonomy, beneficence, non-maleficence, and justice (Beauchamp & Childress, 2009). These four tenets of the principlism approach in medical ethics appear to be very well applicable to emerging neurotechnology (Brukamp, 2010).

The individual patient exercises his right to *autonomy*. *Beneficence* and *non-maleficence* are insofar related as they both stem from the perspective of an external, caring entity that seeks to minimize harm and maximize benefit to the individual. *Justice* is oftentimes applied from a standpoint above the individual, from a level of society, where all goods are supposed to be distributed according to just principles.

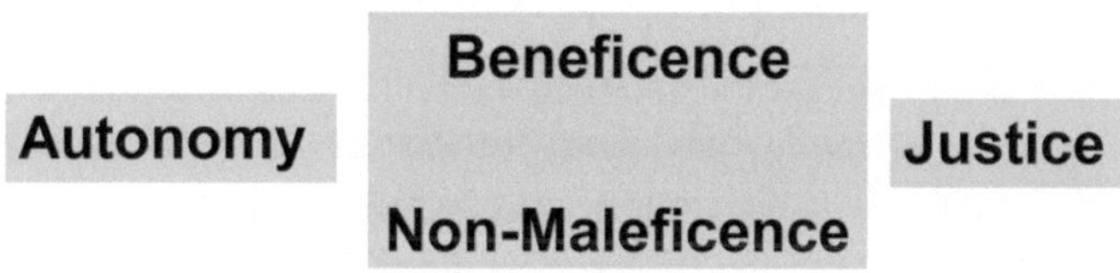

Fig. 6. The four principles in the principlism approach within medical ethics.

The principle of *autonomy* suggests enabling patients to exercise independence in their decision-making. They have to give their informed consent to any medical measure: First, patients are supposed to receive information about their conditions and treatment options, and this information needs to be tailored to their level of understanding. Second, they are to weigh the possibilities themselves and decide about the course of action that suits them best.

Beneficence in the medical realm means to look out for and foster the benefit of patients or subjects. It may encompass supporting the development of devices to aid humans and acquiring evidence for their efficiency. Obviously, beneficence implies that technology, which helps humans, is backed in a number of ways, be it concerning research, development, production, accessibility, and distribution. Medical devices also need to be tested for efficiency according to the approved standards of evidence-based medicine (Sackett et al., 1996). Also, therapies are becoming more and more personalized, a trend that will likely grow in the future. This way, the therapy and enhancement strategies best suited for patients and subjects can be chosen out of a whole array of possibilities.

Non-maleficence, as a principle in medical ethics, asks for a relative absence of negative side effects in relationship to the expected benefits. For example, a treatment with fewer side effects is preferable to one with more when both have the same efficacy. The traditional gold standard is an important guideline for comparison. The side effects need to be assessed in relation to the benefits: Patients may prefer therapies that improve survival with more extensive side effects to those that only work on symptoms with less side effects.

Distributive *justice* means that there is a kind of justified distribution of goods in society. This principle requires competent applications to specific situations. Theories of justice are wide, varied, and heterogeneous, and it therefore defies a brief, comprehensive discussion.

Enhancement partially transcends medicine and is therefore subject to a distinct assessment. Nevertheless, enhancement falls under the extended realm of medical ethics so that the principlism approach still applies:

First, neuroenhancement concerns the *human being as a biological entity*. It alters the physiological functions to achieve something unknown and unprecedented. Therefore, those principles from medical ethics apply that are relevant for the human as a biological entity.

Second, the experts, who assist in the transformation, are the same in medical treatment and medical enhancement: For example, *physicians' expertise* is needed to safely develop and apply new medications, interventions, and technologies. Since enhancement falls under the responsibility of medical providers, the normative principles from medical law and medical ethics apply by extension.

Accordingly, applying the four principles from medical ethics yields the following perspectives and arguments, among others (Brukamp, 2010):

Beneficence and non-maleficence may help to decide between *different categories* of neuroenhancement, namely pharmacological and technological ones. These strategies have diverse side effect profiles. Local treatments, instead of pharmacological ones, may sometimes meanless systemic side effects for the body. Conversely, pharmacological treatments can better be titrated, and increasing knowledge in cell and molecular biology might enable greater insights into mechanisms and eventually more specific treatments with medication. The number of options makes it possible to personalize the enhancement to individual needs. As a general rule, non-invasive measures are preferable to invasive ones because of a more moderate side effect profile.

The steering of technological aids by neural signals, as one example of a potential future application in both neuromedicine and neuroenhancement, requires the acquisition of large amounts of digital data. According to the value of *privacy*, backed by the principles of autonomy, beneficence, and non-maleficence, such data should be utilized only for the benefit of the patients with their informed consent. Confidentiality in this context extends not only to the medical personnel, but to all people who come into contact with the data. This tenet becomes more difficult to be reinforced outside the medical field proper: Confidentiality has a tradition in professional contexts such as medicine, psychology, law, and theology, but its implications are less well known to other fields and the general public.

The principle of justice entails that financial, time, personnel, and other *resources in the health care system* should not be diverted away from those who deserve them most. Therapies were developed to help the sick, disabled, and disadvantaged. Therefore, it would be wrong to strain the infrastructure and the resources of the medical system with the desires of too many clients who ask for enhancements.

6. Ethical assessment of neuroenhancement

Applying the prominent four principles (Beauchamp & Childress, 2009) is one approach of addressing problems in medical ethics. Nevertheless, pro and con arguments may alternatively and more conveniently be grouped according to central topics, which seem to be defining features for the field in question. Accordingly, the current problems of pharmacological neuroenhancement, which extend, in part, to all types of potential future neuroenhancement, can be discussed along the issues of medical risk, lack of evidence, human nature, and justice.

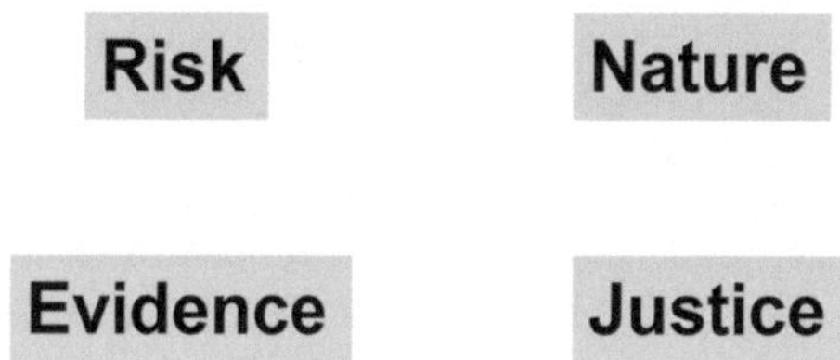

Fig. 7. For an overall assessment of neuroenhancement, there should be, among others, a consideration of medical risk, medical evidence, human nature, and distributive justice. The former two still belong to the narrower realm of responsibility for the field of medicine, whereas the arguments regarding the latter are derived from philosophical theory.

Pharmacological neuroenhancers carry several *medical risks* with them (Banjo et al., 2010): They have side effects, there is a risk of addiction, and they may lose efficacy over time so that higher doses or drug combinations lead to even more risks. In addition, the medications may result in a wrongful subjective overestimation of one's abilities, e.g. regarding attention and insomnia while driving in traffic, which can endanger oneself and others. In most cases, the long-term effects in the healthy population have simply not been studied and are unknown.

The *scientific and medical evidence* that pharmacological neuroenhancers reliably work as expected is scarce. Reviews of the available data show that methylphenidate and modafinil can be said to exhibit some desired effects on healthy people, but may also lead to dangerous overconfidence in one's possibilities (Repantis et al., 2010). Importantly, the end points for potential studies that test neuroenhancers have not been adequately defined: Which ones would be truly deserving and valid end points? They should extend beyond short-term effects and be compatible with other goals that humans have in life. Once these end points are defined, high-quality studies then need to prove the efficacy of the neuroenhancers to achieve them, according to the standards of evidence-based medicine (Sackett et al., 1996).

Humans normally value truth, authenticity, and personal identity (The President's Council on Bioethics, 2003). Some opponents to neuroenhancement regard artificial means for enhancements as (self-)deception and as a threat to *human nature*. Nevertheless, humans have always tried to use tools and to embellish themselves by socially accepted external means - this seems to be a feature of human nature itself. Consequently, the reference to human nature is not one that helps to decide easily between appropriate and inappropriate means of self-improvement; rather, it needs to be applied aptly to different contexts (Groß, 2007a, 2007b).

Supporters of neuroenhancement frequently argue that behavioral modifications have always been employed to achieve the same goals that neuroenhancement serves (Greely et al., 2008) - for example, measures like classic learning and psychotherapy have widely been accepted as valid means. These proponents do not admit that a clear-cut boundary exists between the traditional methods for self-improvement and the novel prospects of neuroenhancement. Nevertheless, such distinctive features of the latter are indeed present and discernible: Medical risks are higher, due to more direct alterations in the brain by medication use or invasive measures; procedures deemed artificial can result in feelings of external determination and self-alienation; effects may suddenly cease secondary to a lack of access to medication or because of technological malfunction, which may be immediate and unforeseeable phenomena.

Considerations from *justice* concern access and coercion. While neuroenhancement may serve the purpose of creating a level playing field for naturally disadvantaged people, performance gaps between groups may widen because of unequal access to the supposedly enhancing medication. Moreover, vulnerable groups, such as children, could experience peer pressure in favor of drug use. Due to their vulnerability, for example because of ongoing brain development, the negative side effects may actually become more extensive.

In summary, a number of arguments caution against the use of neuroenhancement, in particular of the pharmacological variety in use today. Medical arguments refer to risks from medication side effects and from overestimations of one's own abilities, which may become dangerous for oneself and others. Besides, the current evidence for the efficacy of neuroenhancers, aside from short-term effects of some, is thin. While human beings possess a desire for enhancements, not all types are considered compatible with the development and protection of human nature and identity. Enhancement in general may divert resources away from the classic medical system, constituting a challenge to the principle of distributive justice (Racine & Forlini, 2009). Sociological arguments claim that equal access to enhancement routes cannot be guaranteed, and coercion may result in ill effects, particularly in vulnerable groups who cannot decide for themselves, like children.

7. Conclusion

In conclusion, neuroenhancement poses problems due to its nature as a novel enhancement method and because it concerns an organ that mediates human identity. While it cannot be ruled out that acceptable and affordable means may be developed in the future, the long-term benefits cannot easily be foreseen at this time, both on the individual level and from the perspective of society as a whole. Therefore, the best advice is a cautious approach, and the current situation warrants an overall precautionary stance towards neuroenhancement.

8. Acknowledgements

This paper was in part supported by the project "AC-TEC: Gender-Related Acceptance, Usability, and Ethics in New (Medical) Technologies" of the "Exploratory Research

Space@Aachen (ERS)" as part of the German "Exzellenzinitiative des Bundes und der Länder" ("Excellence Initiative"), funded by the "Deutsche Forschungsgemeinschaft (DFG)" ("German Research Foundation").

9. References

Banjo, O.C.; Nadler, R., & Reiner, P.B. (2010). Physician attitudes towards pharmacological cognitive enhancement: safety concerns are paramount. *PLoS ONE* Vol. 5 No. 12, pp. e14322

Beauchamp, T.L., & Childress, J.F. (2009). *Principles of biomedical ethics*, Oxford University Press, New York / Oxford

Brukamp, K. (2010). Aspekte zur medizinethischen Beurteilung von inkorporierter Technologie im Bereich des Gehirns [Aspects of medical ethics to assess internal technology in the brain], In: *Akzeptanz, Nutzungsbarrieren und ethische Implikationen neuer Medizintechnologien: die Anwendungsfelder Telemedizin und Inkorporierte Technik. [Acceptance, barriers to use, and ethical implications of new medical technologies: applications in telemedicine and internal techniques]*, Groß, D.; Gründer, G., & Simonovic, V. (Eds.), pp. 119-124, Kassel University Press, Kassel

Deep-Brain Stimulation for Parkinson's Disease Study Group. (2001). Deep-brain stimulation of the subthalamic nucleus or the pars interna of the globus pallidus in Parkinson's disease. *New England Journal of Medicine*, Vol. 345, No. 13, pp. 956–963

Greely, H.; Sahakian, B.; Harris, J.; Kessler, R.C.; Gazzaniga, M.; Campbell, P., & Farah, M.J. (2008). Towards responsible use of cognitive-enhancing drugs by the healthy. *Nature* Vol. 456, pp. 702–705

Groß, D. (2007a). Neurobionisches und psychopharmakologisches Enhancement - Teil 1: Definitionen, Einsatzbereiche und gesellschaftliche (Vor-)Urteile [Neurobionic and psychopharmacological enhancement - part 1: definitions, areas of use, and judgments and biases in society], In: *Sind die Gedanken frei? Die Neurowissenschaften in Geschichte und Gegenwart [Are thoughts free? The neurosciences in history and present]*, Groß, D., & Müller, S. (Eds.), pp. 216–241, Medizinisch Wissenschaftliche Verlagsgesellschaft, Berlin

Groß, D. (2007b). Neurobionisches und psychopharmakologisches Enhancement - Teil 2: Medizinethische Anmerkungen zu einer aktuellen Debatte [Neurobionic and psychopharmacological enhancement - part 2: remarks from medical ethics on a contemporary debate], In: *Sind die Gedanken frei? Die Neurowissenschaften in Geschichte und Gegenwart [Are thoughts free? The neurosciences in history and present]*, Groß, D., & Müller, S. (Eds.), pp. 242–252, Medizinisch Wissenschaftliche Verlagsgesellschaft, Berlin

Groß, D. (2009a). Blessing or curse? Neurocognitive enhancement by "brain engineering". *Medicine Studies* Vol. 1, No. 4, pp. 379-391

Groß, D. (2009b). Neurobionik und neurobionisches Enhancement - Eine Technik der Zukunft? [Neurobionics and neurobionic enhancement - a technique of the future?], In: *Chancen und Risiken der Neurowissenschaften [Chances and risks of the neurosciences]*, Müller, S.; Zaracko, A.; Groß, D., & Schmitz, D. (Eds.), pp. 74–78, Lehmanns Media, Berlin

Groß, D. (2011). Traditional vs. modern neuroenhancement: notes from a medico-ethical and societal perspective, In: *Implanted minds: the neuroethics of intracerebral stem cell transplantation and deep brain stimulation*, Fangerau, H.; Fegert, J.M, & Trapp, T. (Eds.), pp. 291-311, Transcript, Bielefeld

Hall, W. (2006). Feeling "better than well". *EMBO Reports* Vol. 5, pp. 1105-1109

Hochberg, L.R.; Serruya, M.D.; Friehs, G.M.; Mukand, J.A.; Saleh, M.; Caplan, A.H.; Branner, A.; Chen, D.; Penn, R.D., & Donoghue, J.P. (2006). Neuronal ensemble control of prosthetic devices by a human with tetraplegia. *Nature* Vol. 442, No. 7099, pp. 164-171

Monti, M.M.; Vanhaudenhuyse, A.; Coleman, M.R.; Boly, M.; Pickard, J.D.; Tshibanda, L; Owen, A.M., & Laureys, S. (2010). Willful modulation of brain activity in disorders of consciousness. *New England Journal of Medicine* Vol. 362, No. 7, pp. 579-589

Müller, S., & Christen, M. (2011). Deep brain stimulation in Parkinsonian patients - Ethical evaluation of cognitive, affective, and behavioral sequelae. *AJOB Neuroscience* Vol. 2, No. 1, pp. 3-13

Racine, E., & Forlini, C. (2009). Expectations regarding cognitive enhancement create substantial challenges. *Journal of Medical Ethics* Vol. 35, pp. 469-470

Repantis, D.; Schlattmann, P.; Laisney, O., & Heuser, I. (2010). Modafinil and methylphenidate for neuroenhancement in healthy individuals: a systematic review. *Pharmacological Research* Vol. 62, No. 3, pp. 187-206

Sackett, D.L.; Rosenberg, W.M.; Gray, J.A.; Haynes, R.B., & Richardson, W.S. (1996). Evidence-based medicine: what it is and what it isn't. *British Medical Journal* Vol. 312, No. 7023, pp. 71-72

Talwar, S.K.; Xu, S.; Hawley, E.S.; Weiss, S.A.; Moxon, K.A., & Chapin, J.K. (2002). Rat navigation guided by remote control. *Nature* Vol. 417, No. 6884, pp. 37-38

The President's Council on Bioethics (2003). *Beyond therapy: biotechnology and the pursuit of happiness*, Washington, DC

Velliste, M.; Perel, S.; Spalding, M.C.; Whitford, A.S., & Schwartz, A.B. (2008). Cortical control of a prosthetic arm for self-feeding. *Nature* Vol. 453, No. 7198, pp. 1098-1101.

4

Medical Ethics and Economic Medicalization

Geoffrey Poitras
Faculty of Business Administration,
Simon Fraser University,
Vancouver,
Canada

1. Introduction

Medicalization is typically defined as a societal process where more and more aspects of everyday life come under medical dominion, influence and supervision. The process of medicalization is part of a larger historical transition involving social values associated with traditional institutions, such as the church, the common law and the family, being replaced by the values of science and the scientific method. The practice of medicine has been an important player in this transition. The observation that medicine had "nudged aside" or "replaced" religion as the dominant moral force in the social control of modern societies is a central theme in medicalization research surveyed in the influential review by Conrad (1992). However, the lack of cohesion in this research is reflected in the considerable effort Conrad and others dedicate to the search for a precise definition of 'medicalization'. Writing over a decade later, a continuing lack of cohesion in the state of medicalization research is reflected by Sismondi (2004): "For the most part, medicalization is discussed in terms of the politics of professions, with medical professions gaining importance as they take control over the problems . The means by which economic interests shape medical knowledge and medical discourse have not been well explored"

Recognizing the remarkable technological and economic evolution of the medical profession in the last two decades, Poitras and Meredith (2009), Conrad (2007, 2005) and Conrad and Leiter (2004) find that medicalization is too diverse a concept to be analysed with a unifying methodology. Building on these insights, this chapter explores the analytical advantages of dichotomizing the concept of medicalization into two distinct components: economic medicalization, where the corporate profit motive plays a central role; and, social medicalization, where traditional concerns of social control predominate. Poitras and Meredith (2009) and Poitras (2009) demonstrate that economic medicalization involves a sharp ethical divergence between the goal of shareholder wealth maximization, associated with business ethics, and the norms of science and the scientific method, associated with medical ethics. In turn, the array of substantive global risks associated with the progress of certain elements of modern medical technology makes exploration of the implications of economic medicalization a useful exercise. In this chapter, section 2 details the development of the concept of medicalization, from the early contributions by Szasz and Wootton in the 1950's and continuing to Conrad (2007) and Moloney et al. (2011). Section 3 discusses general differences between: medical ethics, as detailed by the American Medical Association (AMA); and, business ethics, as reflected in the objective of corporate shareholder wealth maximization, e.g., Poitras (1994). Sections 4 and 5 examine two key practical outcomes of economic medicalization: direct-to-consumer marketing of pharmaceuticals; and, medical research that produces ethically questionable outcomes. Finally, the paper concludes with section 6 that considers currently observable trends in economic medicalization.

2. The concept of medicalization[1]

The modern concept of medicalization emerged during the 1950's when Thomas Szasz (born 1920), Barbara Wootton (1897-1988) and others attacked the advance of psychiatry beyond the treatment of well defined mental disorders into areas of dysfunctional behaviour related to crime and delinquency (Wootton 1959; Szasz 1958, 1958a, 1961). These seminal contributions built on Parsons (1951) where the identification of medicine as an institution of social control was initially proposed. Following Szasz and Wootton, 'science' was and is replacing traditional areas of social morality as the means of distinguishing the "undeniably mad" from those "who are simply unable to manage their lives" (Davis 2006, p.51). Yet, the distinction between 'mentally incompetent' and 'sinful' needs to be determined by social values. Allowing 'medical science' to encroach on this decision shifts attention to the individual rather than the environment as the source of the problem. Wootton observes: "Always it is easier to put up a clinic than to pull down a slum." While insightful, the early contributions by Szasz and Wootton only examined the narrow confines of psychiatry where the social implications of medicalization were readily discernible. The extension of these initial notions to a wider field of applications was proposed by Freidson and Zola during the 1970's where the connection between medicalization and social control was more firmly established (Freidson 1970; Zola 1972).

In traditional sociology where social control is a central concept, the connection between social control and medicalization is appealing. The observation that medicine had "nudged aside" or "replaced" religion as the dominant moral force in the social control of modern societies was a central theme in medicalization research surveyed in the influential review by Conrad (1992). However, the lack of cohesion in this research is reflected in the considerable effort Conrad (1992) dedicates to the search for a precise definition of 'medicalization'.[2] Driven by the remarkable evolution of the medical profession in the last

[1] The following discussion updates and extends Poitras (2009).

[2] Writing over a decade later, this lack of cohesion in the state of medicalization research is reflected by Sismondi: "For the most part, medicalization is discussed in terms of the politics of professions, with medical professions gaining importance as they take control over the problems, and sometimes the lives and movements, of a typically disempowered group. Somewhat less frequently, medicalization is discussed in terms of the economics of healthcare industries, including associations of doctors, insurance companies, and drug companies; a few cases include analyses of depression, hyperactivity, osteoporosis, and sexology. The means by which economic interests shape medical knowledge and medical discourse have not been well explored."

two decades, it is becoming gradually apparent that the medicalization concept is too diverse to be analysed with a unifying methodology (Conrad 2007; Conrad and Leiter 2004; Poitras and Meredith 2009). In particular, considerable insight is gained if medicalization is dichotomized into two categories: *social medicalization*, dealing with the type of social control issues that originate with Parsons, Szasz and Wootton; and, *economic medicalization*, dealing with the markets for medical technology and professional services driven by the corporate profit motive.

Defining medicalization as a process where more and more aspects of everyday life come under medical dominion, influence and supervision ultimately requires "the turning of non-medical problems into medical ones" (Sismondi 2004, p.153). Medicalization can occur for various reasons. Drawing a distinction between economic and social medicalization focuses attention on the ethical motives of the medical professionals involved in the process. Social medicalization is concerned with encroachment of the medical profession into areas traditionally controlled by other professions, such as the legal profession for deviant behaviour or the ecclesiastic profession for reproductive decisions. This often leads to a sociological examination of issues surrounding the competition of the professions for social control. While the profit motive may play some role, the complexity of issues surrounding the ethics of the market place are not a central concern. In contrast, economic medicalization encompasses cases where the profit motive plays a substantive role in the transformation of non-medical problems into medical ones. In particular, Healy (2004) identifies economic medicalization with the "marketing of disease".

Numerous instances of economic medicalization have been identified. For example, Conrad and Leiter (2004) examine the direct-to-consumer marketing campaigns by pharmaceutical companies and the development of private medical markets. Conrad (2007) finds evidence of economic medicalization in numerous cases such as: male disorders associated with aging including andropause, baldness and erectile dysfunction; behavioral disorders such as ADHD in adults and hyperactivity in children; and certain applications of biomedical enhancement drugs such as steroids and human growth hormone. Moloney et al. (2010) examine the economic medicalization of sleeplessness. Avorn (2006) details the deceptions pharmaceutical companies have used to hide the evidence of adverse drug effects. Jones and Hagtvelt (2008) consider the tragic implications of treatments for malaria. Instead of seeking the cost-effective solution of eradication by treatment of the local populations, available treatments are targeted at the more profitable Western visitors and ex-patriots sojourning in those regions. In contrast, social medicalization includes studies where the profit motive plays a lesser role, such as studies of spouse battering or gender deviance. The classification of some areas of medicalization research depend on the methodological approach taken, such as studies of childbirth, long term disability, infertility and abortion, where the profit motive may or may not be of central concern.

Since the public policy disasters created by drugs such as elixir sulfanilamide in 1937 and thalidomide in the early 1960's, it has been recognized that medical research and development (R&D) is an area where the conflict of interest between private sector firms guided by the profit motive and those of government acting in the 'public interest' needs to be managed through regulatory oversight. The *raison d'etre* of the institutional review board (IRB) is to ensure that ethical norms of the general population are not put at risk by the private sector firms conducting the bulk of medical R&D that are motivated by the ethical standards of the marketplace. The corporate profit motive provides strong incentives: to recoup R&D expenditures as soon as possible; to recoup acquisition costs related to the takeover of other firms that have developed potentially marketable technologies for drugs or devices; to exploit first mover advantages where the danger of a 'race to market' with potentially competing innovative drugs or devices may be apparent; to develop alternative (off-label) applications and delivery mechanisms for existing drugs; and, to extend drug or device patent protection by reformulations combining these drugs with other existing medications. Faced with a limited time to patent expiration, there is great economic pressure on pharmaceutical companies to move drugs to market as quickly as possible. Rewards are more closely tied to the number of prescriptions written for a drug than to the incremental medical value of the treatment.

The regulatory infrastructure for conducting research through clinical trials is juxtaposed against the corporate requirement of profitability through successful marketing of pharmaceuticals or medical devices. In a world of declining opportunities for highly profitable 'new' patent-able drug discoveries, the stage is set for serious ethical conflict to emerge between the players. This conflict is central to analysis of economic medicalization where the ethical norms of 'science' are confronted with the ethics of the market place, e.g., Angell (2004). In science, accuracy of measurement and validity through replication are fundamental elements. In contrast, the objective of profitability is supported by research, biased or unbiased, that recommends prescription of the treatment on offer. Examples of such bias are accumulating. For example, Heres et al. (2006) examines 33 company sponsored studies of second generation anti-psychotic drugs and finds that in 'head to head' studies involving competing products, the reported total outcome was in favour of the sponsor's drug 90% of the time (Heres et al. 2006, Bhandari et al., 2004). Such an 'empirical' result seems outside the bounds of scientific credibility.

3. Medical ethics and business ethics

Practical examples of the medical profession extending authority over matters not directly concerned with the analysis and treatment of biophysical disorders are readily available. Ethical analysis of such developments is complicated because the 'medical profession' includes not only practising doctors and associations of doctors but also: the pharmaceutical and medical device industry, providing the drugs and medical technologies that are an essential component of modern medicine; the academic institutions and journals involved in training doctors and sponsoring essential research activities; the medical insurance industry that processes payments for the bulk of medical services; and, the government granting agencies and other sponsors that supply essential funding to the research conducted by the medical profession. In addition, governments also play differing roles as medical insurer and provider of medical services, e.g., in Canada the monopoly provider of health services is the federal and provincial governments. Significantly, because the source of capital for the corporations producing pharmaceutical and medical devices is the global financial markets, the primary motivation of these important players in the medical profession differs from those of the other players. The implications of this difference are reflected in the legion of studies on the marketing networks of the pharmaceutical companies and the sophisticated efforts involved in selling products. The differing motivations within the medical profession create a range of potential ethical quandaries.

Due to the diverse and competing ethical norms that impact the medical profession, it is not easy to discern the *de facto* objectives driving particular actions and outcomes. As Poitras and Meredith (2009) observe: "There is an ethical transparency problem". The difficulty of discerning the ethical motivations of specific players within the medical profession can even occur for physicians where the ethics of professional fiduciary responsibility would seem to be clear cut, based on ethical standards stretching back to the Oath of Hippocrates which first appeared around the fifth century B.C., e.g., AMA (2010, p.ix). The Oath protects the rights of the patient by appealing to the strong character of the physician, no formal sanctions or penalties are contemplated. The Oath was "Christianized" around the eleventh century A.D. and remains an essential component of the ideal ethical conduct of physicians up to the present. The evolution of medical practice gradually surpassed the ethical guidance provided by the Oath. Building on contributions from the Scottish physician John Gregory (1724-1773), in 1803 the English physician Thomas Percival (1740-1804) published a 'Code of Medical Ethics' to address the need for more detailed ethical guidance. The Percival code was, more-or-less, adopted by the AMA in 1847 (McCollough 1988). Since that time, a number of major revisions to the Code have been made, with four such revisions during the twentieth century (1903, 1912, 1947, and 1994).[3]

In addition to specifying nine principles of medical ethics, the AMA provides detailed opinions on ethical behaviour for specific situations, e.g., conflicts of interest in biomedical research (AMA 2010).[4] Ethical opinions for over 200 situational problems are currently provided. Opinions cover a wide range of subjects, from the controversial to the mundane. In the realm of social policy, controversial issues such as cloning, euthanasia and gene therapy are examined. More mundane opinions cover inter-professional and hospital relationships and patient confidentiality. Though the present code and related opinions have evolved considerably from the early beginnings of the Oath and the Percival code, basic principles still remain: physicians should base clinical practice and research on the best

[3] The nine principles of the AMA code are (AMA 2010, p.xv): "I. A physician shall be dedicated to providing competent medical care, with compassion and respect for human dignity and rights. II. A physician shall uphold the standards of professionalism, be honest in all professional interactions, and strive to report physicians deficient in character or competence, or engaging in fraud or deception, to appropriate entities. III. A physician shall respect the law and also recognize a responsibility to seek changes in those requirements which are contrary to the best interests of the patient. IV. A physician shall respect the rights of patients, colleagues, and other health professionals, and shall safeguard patient confidences and privacy within the constraints of the law. V. A physician shall continue to study, apply, and advance scientific knowledge, maintain a commitment to medical education, make relevant information available to patients, colleagues, and the public, obtain consultation, and use the talents of other health professionals when indicated. VI. A physician shall, in the provision of appropriate patient care, except in emergencies, be free to choose whom to serve, with whom to associate, and the environment in which to provide medical care. VII. A physician shall recognize a responsibility to participate in activities contributing to the improvement of the community and the betterment of public health. VIII. A physician shall, while caring for a patient, regard responsibility to the patient as paramount. IX. A physician shall support access to medical care for all people."

[4] Similar ethical codes and procedures have been established by the medical associations in other countries, e.g., the code of ethics of the Canadian Medical Association is similar to that of the AMA.

science available; individual self-interest is secondary to the well being of the patient; and, medical knowledge is a public trust to be used to the benefit of patients and society. Significantly, "Principles adopted by the American Medical Association are not laws, but standards of conduct which define the essentials of honorable behavior for the physician" (AMA 2010, p.xvi).

For physicians and other medical professionals engaged in medical research, there are related ethical standards that also apply. Following Weijer et al. (1997): "Medical research involving human subjects raises complex ethical, legal and social issues. Investigators sometimes find that their obligations with respect to a research project come into conflict with their obligations to individual patients." In addition to the AMA code and related opinions, ethical standards for medical research have been set out by a variety of government deparments, agencies and commissions such as the National Commission for the Protection of Human Subjects of Biomedical and Behavioral Research (NCPHS), US Department of Health and Human Services and, in Canada, the Tri-Council of research funding agencies. Medical professionals may also be members of non-governmental organizations that issue statements of ethical standards such as the Council for International Organizations of Medical Sciences and the Human Genome Organization. Recognizing there is some variation in the specific ethical statements, the range of standards proposed for medical research can be roughly and briefly summarized as: obtain informed consent; protect the privacy of patient medical information; and, do no harm.

The long established field of traditional medical ethics is patient centered. While the AMA aims to provide guidance to physicians for dealing with the increasingly complex ethical issues raised by the relentless progress of modern biotechnology, the AMA 'Code of Medical Ethics' is not able to provide sufficient guidance to deal with the multitude of inter-disciplinary ethical problems raised by research into areas such as: cloning; stem cells; genetic modification of foods; euthanasia; DNA data banking; genetic manipulation of human DNA; and, testing for genetic markers. The issues involved are so varied and significant that the field of bioethics has emerged to address such issues, e.g., Eaton (2004). Biotechnology has also impacted research areas that have long-standing social and religious significance such as abortion and the determination of death. While medical ethics has considerable interest in such issues, bioethics goes beyond medical ethics to incorporate knowledge from moral philosophy, law, sociology, molecular biology, economics and other subjects. Central to the issues confronting bioethics is the justification for introducing new technologies. In practice, this ethical problem is confounded by the commercial aspects involved in developing these technologies. The substantial capital investments required for biotechnology advances dictate that bioethics also address the implications of corporate decision making.

Because some of the largest multinational corporations in the world are directly involved in the market for medical products and services, bioethics needs to incorporate elements of business ethics in order to accurately assess a range of important issues. In business ethics it is necessary to recognize that corporations pursue strategies consistent with shareholder wealth maximization (SWM). Following Poitras (1994), the goal of SWM depends on the future common stock price and, as such, does not have ethical transparency. Some assumption about the efficiency of the stock market in valuing ethical concerns is required.

In this vein, the layers of regulatory oversight aimed to restrict unfettered corporate activity come into play. In the key area of medical research, this oversight includes the ethical approval process for medical research in the US embodied in Title 45 Code of Federal Regulation (CFR) Part 46 that empowers the IRB.[5] Similar bodies are empowered in other countries, such as Research Ethics Board (REB) in Canada, e.g., Meredith and Poitras (2008). Also important in the US is Title 21 CFR, Part 56 that requires IRB's to oversee clinical trials of drugs involved in new drug applications to the FDA. Ultimately, it is difficult to expect much more than an 'ethical-is-legal' approach to corporate decisions regarding medical research and development if SWM is the goal. Significantly higher ethical standards may come at a financial cost that impacts corporate profitability undermining achievement of SWM.

In setting the legal and regulatory environment for the medical profession, governments are inclined to adhere to utilitarian ethics where decisions are made on the basis of cost-benefit calculations. The precise method of determining costs and benefits can depend on a range of political and social factors, not just a dollar and cents calculation. The history of tragic events such as the more than 100 deaths associated with the 1937 elixir sulfanilamide incident that gave impetus to the Federal Food, Drug, and Cosmetic Act (1938) and the infamous 1957-61 thalidomide tragedy suggests that crisis management is the primary motivation for substantive changes in the legal and regulatory framework. In contrast to the well established code of medical ethics, the legal environment is a myriad of legislation established at different times with potentially competing ethical standards. In turn, relevant legislation will vary from issue to issue. For example, in the area of direct-to-consumer marketing of genetic tests, regulatory oversight and associated legislation in the US would include: the Federal Trade Commission, the Centers for Disease Control, the Food and Drug Administration and the state health agencies (Berg and Fryer-Edwards 2008, p.27). Similarly, the "Common Rule" principles that inform the institutional process for ethical approval of medical research as reflected in Title 45 CFR apply to some seventeen federal agencies (White 2007).

---

[5] In the US, the 'institutional review board' (IRB) is also referred to with similar names such as the 'independent ethics committee' or 'ethical review board'. The purpose of the IRB is to approve, monitor, and review biomedical and behavioral research involving humans. The primary motivation of IRB activities is to protect the rights and welfare of the human subjects involved in the trial. The legal authority for the IRB can be found in the legislation empowering the Food and Drug Administration (FDA) and Department of Health and Human Services (HHS), It is the HHS regulations that specifically empower IRB's to approve, require modifications in (to secure approval), or disapprove R&D clinical trials. IRB's are governed by the Research Act of 1974, Title 45 CFR (Code of Federal Regulations) part 46. This legislation defines IRB's and requires that IRB's approve all research that receives funding, directly or indirectly, from HHS. Oversight of IRB's resides with the Office for Human Research Protection (OHRP) within HHS. For present purposes, Title 21 CFR, part 56 is also important as this requires IRB's to oversee clinical trials of drugs involved in new drug applications to the FDA. In Canada, the regulatory authority for ethical issues under the Food and Drug Act resides with the "Review Ethics Board" (REB) which is a similar counterpart to the US IRB. The REB's represent the major health catchment regions across the country. Under the Act, REB approval is required to carry out clinical trials involving humans. The corporations seeking approval from an IRB, REB or other such entity in other jurisdictions are, in most cases, multinationals that are involved in acquiring government approval to market patent protected drugs in a number of legal jurisdictions.

4. Direct-to-consumer and direct-to-physician marketing

Economic medicalization is evident in the direct-to-consumer television marketing campaigns by the pharmaceutical companies. Campaigns are designed to put in place a public perception of illness and health consistent with the portfolio of prescription drug products on offer, e.g., Moynihan and Cassels (2005); Brennan et al. (2010). Where bodies were once understood as normatively healthy and only sometimes ill, effective marketing has individuals seeing their bodies as inherently ill, and only able to be brought towards health with the effective medical treatment. The history of Viagra and the erectile dysfunction drugs attest to the ability of the direct-to-consumer marketing by pharmaceutical companies to transform a non-medical problem into a medical one. The treatment of risk factors for illness and not just the associated illness has also allowed pharmaceutical companies to dramatically increase the sales of prescription drugs. Other instances of the types of drugs that have exhibited substantial direct-to-consumer promotional spending are anti-psychotic agents, proton pump inhibitors, COX-2 inhibitors and HMG-CoA reductase inhibitors (Donohue et al. 2007, p.677). Given the difficulty of determining whether a good outcome has resulted from the perceived 'risk' being successfully treated, this is a potentially much more profitable area for pharmaceutical company marketing campaigns to pursue than the development of drugs that treat actual diseases.

Economic medicalization involves a complicated web of interaction between physicians, responsible for prescribing drugs and delivering medical care, and the pharmaceutical and medical device companies that supply the products that are essential to the practice of modern medicine. Rules on direct-to-consumer marketing vary across jurisdictions and medical products. For example, regulatory oversight of the direct-to-consumer marketing of genetic testing kits in the US would involve the Federal Trade Commission, the Centers for Disease Control, the Food and Drug Administration and the state health agencies (Berg and Fryer-Edwards 2008, p.27). In the realm of direct-to-consumer marketing, only the US and New Zealand currently leave this marketing method largely unrestricted. Other countries, such as Canada, allow such marketing with relatively lenient restrictions and may reduce restrictions further in the future (Cassels 2006). In the US, direct-to-consumer marketing was permitted through a regulatory decision of the FDA in 1998. Pines (1999) provides an historical overview of direct-to-consumer advertising up to the administrative change in FDA rules.

Examining the marketing methods that companies use to influence treatment selection assists in identifying sources of ethical conflict in the medical R&D process. Following Donohue et al. (2007, p.676), spending on advertising and promotion to medical professionals and consumers in 2005 was: $4.2 billion for direct-to-consumer advertising; $18.4 billion for free samples mostly given to physicians; $6.8 billion for detailing; and, $429 million for journal advertising. One key marketing strategy revolves around influencing the opinion leaders.[6] Applying this strategy to the case of medical drugs and devices, opinion leaders can be identified with groups such as specialists, research faculty, heavy prescribers in a drug/device category and product champions. Considerable effort is given to finding

[6] The following discussion relies on Poitras and Meredith (2009).

opinion leaders willing to speak favourably about a company's product. In many cases, opinion leaders derive financial gain from interacting with medical product marketers at a number of levels. Marketers try to influence opinion leaders because these groups, in turn, affect the purchasing habits of other buyers who respect the opinion leaders' knowledge base and authority in a particular area. Following Poitras and Meredith (2009), the lack of "ethical transparency" in the motivations of opinion leaders in this process raises a number of ethical issues.

The points of interaction between opinion leaders in the medical profession and companies marketing medical goods and services are numerous. Opinion leaders are retained: to provide presentations regarding research results at various venues; deliver lectures at conferences financed in whole or in part by the corporations that retain the opinion leader; acting as paid consultants to those corporations; and, offering symposia for continuing medical education in their fields of expertise. Such interactions, which are also arguably the legitimate business of the participants, cause ethical concern when it is difficult to determine the degree of independence that the opinion leaders are able to exercise given the financial and personal relationships that have developed between themselves and the corporations with whom they interact. Concerns arise that these 'relationship marketing' strategies may positively influence physician perceptions of the corporation and the products on offer, e.g., in qualitative evaluations of drug efficacy. The extent of this marketing strategy is somewhat staggering. Excluding free drug samples, Campbell (2007) estimates that 78% of U.S. physicians have been financially involved with industry: 35% received reimbursements; 18% were paid for consultancy; 16% had funded speaking engagements; 9% served on advisory boards; and, 3% were involved in clinical trials recruitment.

While it is tempting to conclude that opinion leaders are of sufficient ethical stature that actual and substantive knowledge of the subject will dictate an unbiased reading of the evidence, it is not always clear whether published research by a given opinion leader is free from the influence of economic medicalization. In particular, 'ghost-writing' is a marketing/research strategy where a drug company will carry out research and then forward the manuscript to an author in attempt to secure their endorsement. Obviously, only those research results favourable to the product are forwarded to the prospective author. By attaching a respected author's name to the research results, the company hopes to achieve more rapid acceptance of the drug or device in the marketplace than if the product was only advertised (Healy 2004). This strategy is particularly attractive to academic research faculty where publications in prestigious journals have considerable value to career progress. In turn, ghost-written and other positive published research permits sales representatives of a drug or medical device company to bring these trial results to the prescribing physician in an effort to influence prescription pattern choices.

While the enlistment of opinion leaders plays a fundamental role in corporate marketing strategies, it is has traditionally been the prescribing physician that drug companies need to influence the most. Though this approach has changed somewhat with the rise of direct-to-consumer marketing, the bulk of advertising and promotion spending is still targeted directly at physicians. A key element in this strategy is the 'detail man'. It is estimated that there is approximately one pharmaceutical company sales representative for every 10 doctors in most developed countries. The history of the modern detail man can be traced back to the 1940-1960 era when the prescription drug industry was in a period of enormous expansion (Greene 2004). To address the dramatic changes in the medical profession brought on by the advent of a host of new and important prescription drugs, detail men during the period were transformed "from specialized salesmen into quasi-professionals". The pharmaceutical companies recognized the value to drug sales if detail men could be seen as assistants to doctors, conveying useful information about important drug developments rather than being a mere salesman for products. Greene (2004) argues that this change of image "required a careful negotiation around doctors' spaces, both figuratively and literally."

The lack of ethical transparency in the activities of detail men is apparent (Poitras and Meredith 2009). Though detail men can not be seen as telling doctors what to prescribe, their role is ultimately to influence prescription behaviours. To do this, detail men want to be seen by physicians as allied professionals, consciously modelled as having the same ethical objectives as doctors. For example, Greene (2004) reports that manuals for detail men reproduce parts of the AMA's code of ethics. To be effective, detail men need to have the ability to interact with doctors, and require training to develop this ability. Detailing has to at least appear to educate, rather than merely to sell. In this process, the research pipeline of positive results are an invaluable tool for the detail men. Marketing to doctors often takes the form of getting doctors up to speed on the latest research. The range of techniques that can accomplish this goal includes not only marketing by pharmaceutical representatives, but also advertisements in professional journals, funding continuing medical education conferences and so on.

Given that drug detailing and sampling are based on the marketing tactics used to generate demand for any product, not just pharmaceuticals and medical devices, the suspicion of economic medicalization is difficult to displace. Drug and medical device sales representatives bring research literature and clinical trial results to the doctors in efforts to influence prescription pattern choices, while at the same time company funded research ensures that unsuccessful clinical trials not get published so physicians are exposed mainly to studies supportive of the drug or medical device (Turner 2008). Influential opinion leaders tend to be involved in the clinical trials that are positively predisposed toward the sponsoring company's drug or medical device (Anderson 2006). This can have a positive affect on the perception of their peers toward the product (Steinman et al. 2006). Sales representatives attempt to influence physicians through 'relationship marketing' where personal interaction with physicians is used to influence decisions. One example of such relationship marketing occurs where company representatives pay 'preceptor fees' (in some cases up to $1000 per day) to accompany surgeons in operating rooms and clinics. While the stated objective is to learn how physicians actually used the drug or medical device, serious concerns for medical ethics are raised regarding the protection of patient confidentiality and the potential for private funds flowing to doctors influencing physician choices of medical products.

A key element in marketing to physicians is the provision of free samples in order to impact on prescription patterns. Chew et al. (2000) conclude that the availability of drug samples led their primary physician respondents to prescribe drugs different from their preferred choice, especially if it avoided costs to the patient. Campbell (2007) in a national U.S. survey reported that 78% of 1,255 physician respondents had received free samples. Pharmaceutical companies do not undertake that level of free sample distribution unless it has a track record of producing results. Marketing research has long established that providing free samples is one of the strongest cues in terms of producing product trial and adoption. Medical product representatives donate substantial quantities of free samples to hospitals and clinics, presumably with the objective of slowly infiltrating the facility and subtly influencing staff usage patterns of drugs, devices and medical supplies. With the goal of promoting product efficacy, drug representatives aim to interact directly with hospital staff instead of, say, working through hospital pharmacologists who possess far greater knowledge of drug efficacy and safety and are much better equipped to evaluate drug alternatives.

5. Economic medicalization of research studies[7]

The medical research literature abounds with examples of bias in empirical studies of pharmaceutical effectiveness such as: studies with fundamental design flaws where no control groups or placebo arms are involved; and, studies where poor comparators are used, e.g., the sponsored drug is compared to a placebo (no treatment) instead of the most effective comparator drug available (Bero and Rennie 1996). Additional bias can be introduced by the method of comparison used. For example, economic cost comparisons are sometimes avoided when the effectiveness of new experimental drugs is being assessed. Due to large accumulated R&D expenses, such long patent-life drugs can be substantially more expensive than comparable predecessor drugs. Effectiveness measurement could emphasize, say, patient mortality instead of the increase in mortality compared to cheaper generic drugs that have comparable effectiveness. Sample bias can also be compromised through the impact of study entry criteria, such as excluding pregnant women or restricting ethnic minorities into the sample population.

Economic medicalization of research studies is a process where the traditional values associated with the scientific method are replaced by research ethics that reflect the values of the market place. While traditional scientific values demand the researcher be as objective as possible in order to reduce the possibility of bias in the interpretation of the observed data, the ethics of the marketplace are more concerned with abnormal gains (losses) associated with 'positive' (negative) research results. In statistical terms, economic medicalization occurs when there is a decided bias towards unjust acceptance and against unjust rejection. One documented instance where this occurs is 'publication bias': a tendency to publish only favourable clinical trial results of an experimental drug. Corporate sponsors have little interest in providing negative information regarding a product in which they may have already invested millions of dollars. Even journal editors may show a predilection for publishing successful, as opposed to failed, clinical trial results (Schafer 2004). Consequently, the medical community observes the positive research study results for the drug that accumulate in the published literature rather than the failed trials of the drug which languish in the 'file drawer'.

Another instance of economic medicalization is 'muzzle clauses' in the contracts of investigators involved in clinical trials. These clauses are intended to prevent researchers

[7] This section is derived from Meredith and Poitras (2009, sec.3)

from releasing any information about the clinical trial without the sponsor's permission. This can be problematic if the physician discovers significant safety concerns related to the trial. If the researcher releases the negative information, the terms of the muzzle clause are breached and a variety of undesirable outcomes can result. Examples of possible outcomes include: threats of civil lawsuits; the sponsoring company withdrawing financial support for the researcher and, possibly reducing or eliminating philanthropic contributions to the host institution; and, the sponsoring company engaging outside experts to refute the researcher's findings. However, if the researcher sits on the information the doctor-patient accord to act in the best interests of the research subjects recruited for the drug trial is breached. Many facets of muzzle clauses emerged in the the Nancy Olivieri versus Apotex case that received international coverage in medical and ethics journals and is used as a classic example of the failure to deal effectively with the problems posed by restricting negative results from drug trials (Schafer 2004; Somerville 2002; Thompson et al. 2001).

The controversy involving Apotex Inc., Dr. Nancy Olivieri and the Hospital for Sick Children in Toronto (the Hospital) originated in clinical studies of the drug L1 (deferiprone) that generated disputes between Apotex and Dr. Olivieri, between Dr. Olivieri and other investigators and between Dr. Olivieri and the Hospital. L1 was first synthesized in 1987 and a research study by Dr. Olivieri and Dr. Gideon Koren of L1 patients at the Hospital began in 1989, funded by the federal government's Medical Research Council of Canada (MRC). When this funding ended in 1992, an alternative source of funding was received from Apotex. While the company was initially reluctant to get involved with the development of L1 because of its impaired patent status and because it produced serious side-effects in some patients, Apotex ultimately obtained a licence to develop L1 from the patent holder and a drug trial conducted by Olivieri and Koren was sponsored which involved patients with thalassemia major, a disorder that impacts hemoglobin production. Participants in the study were randomly assigned to receive either L1 or deferoxamine, the established treatment for iron toxicity. The randomized trial was constructed to compare the effects of the two drugs on body iron levels. The contract between the researchers and Apotex governing the drug trial contained a muzzle clause.

Details of the subsequent L1 drug trial are well known, e.g., Thompson et al. (2001). There was tension between Dr. Olivieri and officials of Apotex almost from the beginning, at least partly due to differences in expectations between the investigators who viewed the trials as continuing research work done under the MRC grant and Apotex whose expectations were consistent with the usual procedures for the initiation and conduct of industry funded drug studies. While in April 1995, the investigators published a paper indicating a 'favorable effect of deferiprone on iron balance', by the autumn of 1995, some negative data were emerging from the compassionate use trial. This data was seen by Dr. Olivieri as a 'loss of response' or 'loss of efficacy' in some patients receiving L1. Apotex objected to this characterization, interpreting the findings as being due to variability in response that is seen with most drugs. In March 1996, Dr. Olivieri reported her findings of loss of response to the REB for the Hospital and was instructed to modify the patient information and consent forms and to advise physicians treating patients with L1 at other centres of the findings.

In early May 1996, Apotex indicated to the REB that investigators in other centres involved in the drug trial did not agree with Dr. Olivieri's interpretation and that Apotex had convened an expert panel of international stature to review the data. On May 24, 1996, Apotex wrote to Olivieri and Koren informing them that Apotex was not renewing the trials contract which had expired some weeks earlier. In this communication, Apotex reminded the researchers of the contract's confidentiality provision that: "all information whether written or not, obtained or generated by the Investigators during the term of the LA-O1 [randomized trial] Agreement and for a period of one year thereafter, shall be and remain secret and confidential and shall not be disclosed in any manner to any third party except with the prior written consent of Apotex. Please be aware that Apotex will take all possible steps to ensure that these obligations of confidentiality are met and will vigorously pursue all legal remedies in the event there is any breach of these obligations." On the same date, Dr. Olivieri was informed that an additional consulting contract with Apotex would not be renewed and the same warning was issued to her about breaches of its confidentiality provisions.

Needless to say, Olivieri was not deterred by the muzzle clause. In July 1996, the expert panel appointed by Apotex produced a report that supported the Apotex interpretation of the variability in response to L1. Dr. Olivieri produced a commentary rebutting these findings and reaffirming the negative conclusions about the efficacy of L1. Starting in early December 1996, Dr. Olivieri began to disseminate the negative L1 results at a variety of professional conferences including the American Society of Hematology. In the time leading up to these presentations, Apotex indicated repeatedly that the company did not concur in the findings that L1 caused liver fibrosis in some patients and would not consent to the submission of the abstracts for publication. Dr. Olivieri was again notified that she would be breaching the contract if she proceeded to do so. Apotex also questioned the data supporting the conclusion, and arranged to have an independent analysis done by a leading expert on liver pathology. This expert came to a different conclusion than Dr. Olivieri, finding that L1 did not exacerbate liver fibrosis. Much of the subsequent notoriety and public attention the case received was due to the desire of Olivieri to publicize the events.

Muzzle clauses are a relatively obvious implication of economic medicalization. Other implications are less obvious. Consider the issue of drug trial sample design. While concerns of public safety argue for a time series analysis of experimental medical products, economic pressures to bring a drug to market as soon as possible result in cross-sectional static (as opposed to dynamic) analyses. This fosters large Phase 3 trials where sample sizes are substantial, but the elapsed time may be insufficient for dynamic or cumulative effects of the experimental product to emerge. Phase 4 or post-marketing approval trials can be longer term and much more effective at detecting time series based cumulative effects. Yet, there is no requirement that phase 4 post-marketing or tracking studies be conducted or reported. The tragic consequences of OcyContin, Neurontin, Paxil, Accutane, (Caplovitz, 2006) Baycol, Aprotinin and Vioxx (Avorn, 2006) speak clearly to the dangers of long-term cumulative effects that have emerged only after extended periods of time in the market place.

Because present regulations do not require drug and device firms to carry out and publicly vet phase 4 research programs, the law and the ethical issues surrounding Phase 4 clinical research trials are ill defined. A company that is concerned about the longer term side effects of a drug might carry out a longitudinal tracking study as a means of exhibiting due diligence. If negative results are found, the company would arguably have an ethical responsibility to make those side effects known and, if serious enough, voluntarily pull the drug from the market. However, there is evidence that in some serious cases voluntary withdrawal did not happen, a consequence of the desire to avoid the multi-million dollar investment losses for the pharmaceutical company stockholders that can occur when such negative news is released to the capital market (Caplovitz 2006, Avorn 2006). In economic terms, a decision not to withdraw a drug (e.g., Vioxx) has to be weighed off against the danger of civil litigation associated with the damage done by the drug's side effects. This ethical-is-legal conundrum may also lead to effective Phase 4 trials not being carried out since if no negative side effects are found then there is no obligation to report them publicly (Avorn 2006).

6. Future trends in economic medicalization

Recent evidence suggests that a form of economic medicalization is happening in Phase 4 studies. In 2000, Phase 4 studies accounted for 3.1% of all clinical trials worldwide that were registered with the U.S. National Institutes of Health. In 2008, Phase 4 trials accounted for 16.7% of all registered trials, though it is difficult to tell whether this increase was due to the increased registration of Phase 4 trials or to an actual increase in the number of such studies. In this vein, evidence points to the increasing use of primary physicians to conduct Phase 4 trials where remuneration is paid for participation. At this point, it is unclear whether these studies constitute 'real research' with properly structured Phase 4 research protocols that would meet IRB standards or are just disguised 'drug seeding' marketing strategies. Deshpande and El-Chibini (2005) certainly point to the latter hypothesis, providing advice to pharmaceutical companies on how Phase 4 studies can be used to attract physician participation in order to generate new drug sales. This approach appears to be supported by Andersen et al. (2006) where it is reported that when general practitioners were paid $800 US per patient to recruit subjects for an asthma study, there was an increase in the long term use of the trial sponsor's drug.

One disturbing aspect of economic medicalization is the transformation of the process for doing clinical trials into exercises that are motivated more as marketing vehicles than needed R&D. One immediate advantage of such a marketing strategy is that physicians can legitimately receive fees for the recruitment and tracking of subjects admitted into the clinical trials. In some instances these fees are not inconsequential. For example, Sismondi (2004, p.149) describes a US research study by Biovail that paid a fee of $1000 for doctors, plus $150 for office management expenses, for patient data when at least 11 of their patients renewed a prescription to Cardizem, a drug intended for long-term use. In this case, paying doctors to get patients started on a course of treatment could lead to substantial profits from these prescriptions. Doctors who signed up for the trial but did not keep 11 patients on the drug received US$250 for participation. According to ethicists who commented on the case, a US$1000 payment to doctors was unusually high for a post-marketing research trial.

Another ethically disturbing aspect of the evolution of economic medicalization concerns off-label prescription drug usage. The prescription drug approval process is based on research and clinical trials where specific drugs and medical devices are approved by review boards for specific applications. However, once approved, companies have economic incentives to promote use of the drug for other medical conditions without further research reviews by government. Delays in seeking approval for alternative uses are consistent with obtaining a maximum revenue stream for a given product, if only because alternative uses can be a basis for a further round of patent protection. For example, Pfizer admitted guilt in the case of gabapentin (Neurontin), a drug originally intended for the treatment of epilepsy. The company subsequently used opinion leaders to market the drug to physicians for a range of other indications. Steinman et al. (2006) estimate the company spent $40 million U.S. in advertising and promotion with 50-66% of that budget going to professional education between 1996 and 1998. Significantly increased market penetration was achieved by selling gabapentin off-label. In general, Radley et al. (2006) estimate that 21% of all drug use in the U.S. among office based physicians was for off-label indications and that 73% of off-label uses lacked strong scientific evidence.

Discernible trends in the pattern of economic medicalization indicate a number of flash points that threaten to undermine the validity of the present medical R&D clinical trial approval process. Regarding Phase 4 or post-approval research studies, there is currently no requirement that results of such studies need to be released or even that such trials be conducted according to IRB approved protocols. In situations where negative or ineffective results are found, companies will be reluctant to release such results and, without IRB oversight, will not be required to do so. Two particularly egregious cases where this has occurred is Bayer admitting to a 'mistake' in suppressing a study that showed dangerous side-effects associated with the drug Baycol and Merck's suppression of studies that showed Vioxx doubled the risk of myocardial infarction and stroke (Avorn 2006). These studies only came to light because the adverse negative reaction spread over a large population was sufficiently detectable by other means. At present, exact information on the number of unregistered Phase 4 trials is not available, nor is the amount of remuneration flowing to physicians who enroll patients in these 'trials'.

Unfortunately, aiming to increase the reach and depth of ethical oversight in order to prevent questionable research practices may, in the end, be self-defeating. Faced with rising costs associated with obtaining clinical trial approval in developing countries, pharmaceutical companies are moving certain types of medical R&D offshore to third world jurisdictions where the ethical requirements of the drug approval process are substantially less due to lower costs, lax regulations and uneducated research subjects that make for more freedom in research design and lower all-in costs of doing experimental trials (O'Neill 2008). Arguably questionable randomization procedures have been observed in some research protocols used in third world countries. The classic case involved the randomization of African subjects to a placebo arm of a HIV drug study where an existing 'gold standard' treatment was available for comparison. Consequently certain HIV pregnant women received no treatment at all under the placebo arm of the study when a life-saving drug could have been administered without adversely affecting the trial results. Cost effectiveness in medical R&D seems an appropriate iteration on the economic medicalization theme.

A final point of ethical concern can be found in the now rapidly emerging development of private research data bases. Such data bases are being created when clinical trials request subjects give blood and tissue samples for 'future research'. Modern technology permits these samples to be analyzed to the molecular and genetic level and this information entered into the data base. Such requests for blood and tissue samples are now commonplace in the consent forms and clinical trial protocols submitted to IRB's. The data bases are conducive to in-house analysis by pharmaceutical companies. At present, even though the data were obtained from an approved clinical trial, there is no process to ensure that negative findings associated with experimental drugs obtained through exploitation of the data base will be subjected to public scrutiny by the IRB (Avorn 2006). It is fascinating that, as with other areas of marketing research, large data bases appear to have become the currency of R&D in the new millennium. With the rapid development of such large scale data-bases in the last decade, Phase 4 studies can also be conducted in house using multivariate observational analysis, more-or-less ensuring the privacy of the Phase 4 statistical results and avoiding problems of public scrutiny.

7. References

American Medical Association (2010) *Code of Medical Ethics of the American Medical Association, Current Opinions with Annotations 2010-11,* Chicago, IL: American Medical Association.

Andersen, M., J. Kragstrup and J. Sondergaard (2006) 'How Conducting a Clinical Trial Affects Physicians' Guideline Adherence and Drug Preferences', *Journal of the American Medical Association* 295 (June): 2759 - 2764.

Angell, M. (2004) *The Truth About Drug Companies: How They Deceive Us and What To Do About It.* New York: Random House.

Avorn, J. (2006) 'Dangerous Deception' Hiding the Evidence of Adverse Drug Effects', *New England Journal of Medicine* 355 (Nov.): 2169-2171.

Berg, C. and K. Fryer-Edwards (2008) 'The Ethical Challenges of Direct-to-Consumer Genetic Testing', *Journal of Business Ethics* 77: 17-31.

Bero, L. and D. Rennie (1996) 'Influences on the Quality of Published Drug Studies', *International Journal of Technology Assessment in Health Care* 12: 209-237.

Bhandari, M., J. Busse, D. Jackowski, V. Montori, H. Schünemann, S. Sprague, D. Mears, E. Schemitsch, D. Heels-Ansdell and P.J. Devereaux (2004) 'Association Between Industry Funding and Statistically Significant Pro-industry Findings in Medical and Surgical Randomized Trials', *Canadian Medical Association Journal* 170: 477-480.

Brennan, R., L. Eagle and D. Rice (2010) 'Medicalization and Marketing', *Journal of Macromarketing* 30: 8-22.

Campbell, E. (2007) 'Doctors and Drug Companies: Scrutinizing Influential Relationships', *New England Journal of Medicine* 357 (Nov.): 1796-1797.

Canadian Institutes of Health Research, Natural Sciences and Engineering Research Council of Canada, Social Sciences and Humanities Research Council of Canada (1998) *Tri-Council Policy Statement: Ethical Conduct for Research Involving Humans 1998* (with 2000, 2002, 2005 amendments).

Caplovitz, A. (2006) 'Turning Medicine into Snake Oil: How pharmaceutical marketers put patients at risk', *New Jersey Public Interest Research Group Law and Policy Center:* 1-52.

Cassels, A. (2006) 'Canada may be forced to allow direct to consumer advertising', *British Medical Journal* 332: 1469.

Chew, L., T. O'Young, T Hazlet, K Bradley, C. Maynard, and D. Lessler (2000) 'A Physician Survey of the Effect of Drug Sample Availability on Physicians' Behavior', *Journal of General Internal Medicine* 15: 478-483.

Conrad, P. (2007) *The Medicalization of Society*. Baltimore, MD: Johns Hopkins Press.

Conrad, Peter. (2005) 'The Shifting Engines of Medicalization', *Journal of Health and Social Behavior* 46: 3-14.

Conrad, Peter. (1992) 'Medicalization and Social Control', *Annual Review of Sociology* 18, 209-32.

Conrad, Peter and V. Leiter (2004) 'Medicalization, Markets and Consumers', *Journal of Health and Social Behavior* 45 (Supplement): 158-76.

Davis, J. (2006) 'How Medicalization Lost Its Way', *Society* 43: 51-56.

Deshpande, R. and S. El-Chibini (2005) 'Scientific Marketing Offers a New Way to Get Prescribers', *Canadian Pharmaceutical Marketing* (Feb.): 37-38.

Donohue, J., M. Cevasco and M. Rosenthal (2007) 'A Decade of Direct-to-Consumer Advertising of Prescription Drugs', *New England Journal of Medicine* 357 (August 16): 673-681.

Eaton, M. (2004) *Ethics and the Business of Bioscience*, Stanford, CA: Stanford University Press.

Eaton, M. (2008) 'Managing the Risks Associated with using Biomedical Ethics Advice', *Journal of Business Ethics* 77: 99-109.

Freidson, E. (1970) *Profession of Medicine*. New York: Dodd, Mead.

Greene, J. (2004) 'Attention to 'Details': Etiquette and the Pharmaceutical Salesmen in Postwar USA', *Social Studies of Science* 34: 271-92.

Healy, D. (2004) 'Shaping the Intimate: Influences on the Experience of Everyday Nerves', *Social Studies of Science* 34: 219-245.

Heres, S., J. Davis, K. Maino, E. Jetzinger, W. Kissling, and S. Leucht (2004) 'Why Olanzapine Beats Risperidone, Risperidone Beats Quetiapine, and Quetiapine Beats Olanzapine: An Exploratory Analysis of Head-to-Head Comparison Studies of Second-Generation Antipsychotics', *American Journal of Psychiatry* 194: 185-194.

Jones, G. and R. Hagtvedt (2008) 'Marketing in Heterozygous Advantage', *Journal of Business Ethics* 77: 85-87.

Lynch, M. (2004) 'Ghost Writing and Other Matters', *Social Studies of Science* 34: 147-148.

McCullough, L. (1998) *John Gregory and the Invention of Professional Medical Ethics and the Profession of Medicine*, Dordrecht, Netherlands: Kluwer.

Meredith, L. and G. Poitras (2008) 'Ethical Transparency and Government Regulation of Canada's Medical Research Industry', *Forum on Public Policy Online*, (Spring).

Moloney, M., T. Konrad and C. Zimmer (2011) 'The Medicalization of Sleeplessness: A Public Health Concern', *American Journal of Public Health* 101: 1429-1433.

Moynihan, R. and A. Cassels (2005) *Selling sickness: how the world's biggest pharmaceutical companies are turning us all into patients*. Vancouver, BC : Greystone Books.

O'Neil, P. (2008) 'Ethics Guidelines for Clinical Trials to be Revised', *Canadian Medical Association Journal* (Jan.) 15: 138.

Parsons, T. (1951) *The Social System*. New York: Free Press.

Pines, W. (1999) 'A history and perspective of direct-to-consumer marketing', *Food and Drug Law Journal* 54: 489-518.

Poitras, G. and L. Meredith (2009) 'Ethical Transparency and Economic Medicalization', *Journal of Business Ethics* 86: 313-325.

Poitras, G. (2009) "Business Ethics, Medical Ethics and Economic Medicalization" *International Journal of Business Governance and Ethics* 4: 372-89.

Poitras, G. (1994) 'Shareholder Wealth Maximization, Business Ethics and Social Responsibility' *Journal of Business Ethics*. 13: 125-34.

Radley, D., S. Finkelstein and R. Stafford (2006) 'Off-Label Prescribing Among Office based Physicians', *Archives of Internal Medicine* 166: 1021-1026.

Schafer, A. (2004) 'Biomedical Conflicts of Interest: A Defence of the Sequestration Thesis: Learning From the Cases of Nancy Olivieri and David Healy', *Journal of Medical Ethics* 30: 8-24.

Sismondo, S. (2004) 'Pharmaceutical Maneuvers', *Social Studies of Science* 34: 149-159.

Somerville, M. (2002) 'A postmodern moral tale: the ethics of research relationships', *Nature* 1 (April): 316-20.

Steinman, M., L. Bero, M. Chren and S. Landefeld (2006) 'Narrative Review: The Promotion of Gabapentin: An Analysis of Internal Industry Documents', *Annals of Internal Medicine* 145 (August).

Szasz, T. (1958) 'Psychiatry, Ethics, and the Criminal Law', *Columbia Law Review*, 58 (February): 183-198.

Szasz, T.(1958a) 'Scientific Method and Social role in Medicine and Psychiatry', *A.M.A. Archives of Internal Medicine*, 101 (Feb.): 228-238.

Szasz, T. (1961) *The Myth of Mental Illness*, New York: Harper and Row.

Thompson, J., P. Baird and J. Downie (2001) *The Olivieri report : the complete text of the report of the independent inquiry commissioned by the Canadian Association of University Teachers*. Toronto : J. Lorimer.

Turner E., A. Matthews, E. Linardatos, R. Tell, and R. Rosenthal (2008) 'Selective Publication of Antidepressant Trials and Its Influence on Apparent Efficacy', *New England Journal of Medicine* 358: 252-260.

Weijer, C., B. Dickens and E.. Meslin (1997) 'Bioethics for clinicians: 10. Research ethics', *Canadian Medical Association Journa*l 156: 1153-7

White, R. (2007) 'Institutional Review Board Mission Creep: The Common Rule, Social Science and the Nanny State', *The Independent Review* XI (Spring): 547-64.

Wootton, B. (1959) *Social science and social pathology* (assisted by Vera G. Seal and Rosaling Chambers) New York : Macmillan.

Zola, I. (1972) 'Medicine as a institution of social control', *Sociology Review* 20: 487-504.

5

Decision-Making in Neonatology: An Ethical Analysis from the Catholic Perspective

Peter A. Clark
Saint Joseph's University
USA

1. Introduction

Dramatic advances in neonatal medical information and technology occur daily and these advances are being implemented almost immediately. Despite the dramatic technological advances, diagnostic and prognostic certainty for many neonatal conditions remains illusive. As a result, the appropriate decision-makers have to decide whether some handicapped newborns, such as those with congenital anomalies, low-birth-weights, and genetic defects, should be treated aggressively or not at all. This uncertainty has led to many handicapped newborns with serious congenital anomalies being treated aggressively. This treatment prolongs the lives of many newborns when in the past they would have been allowed to die. Such life-prolonging treatment decisions have far-reaching ramifications. One thing that is clear to serious observers in the field is that the implementation of medical advances and technology for some newborns is a mixed blessing at best. Despite proposed federal regulations (1984 Child Abuse Law)[1] and medical guidelines (American Academy of Pediatrics) [2] that have helped to clarify treatment issues, there is still no consensus among responsible decision-makers on a moral criterion to assist parents and health care professionals on treatment decisions. There is general agreement within the medical, legal, and ethical professions that there are some handicapped newborns, in particular situations, whose lives need not be saved. Consensus ends, however, when an attempt is made to determine which specific newborns should receive or not receive medical treatment. This diversity of opinions has brought to the forefront the urgent need for a normative moral criterion to assist decision-makers in their discernment of treatment decisions for these never-competent patients.[3]

Today, parents and health care professionals are often forced to draw lines between newborns who will be treated and those who will not be. If these lines are being drawn, then ethicist Richard A. McCormick argues, "it is of public importance that we find out the criteria by which they are being drawn. My attempt is to search our tradition on the meaning of life and so forth and see if we couldn't develop criteria."[4] Realizing the magnitude of this problem, McCormick has established a moral criterion for treatment decisions regarding handicapped newborns as a revised natural-law ethicist in the Roman Catholic tradition.

As a revised natural-law ethicist, McCormick has always sought a balanced middle course between extreme positions--a course which he understands as characteristic of the Judaeo-

Christian tradition.[5] Few, if any, physicians are willing to make substantive criteria when it comes to treatment decisions for handicapped newborns. On the other hand, moral theologians, in their concern to avoid total normlessness and arbitrariness, can easily become quite dogmatic.[6] Between the two extremes of the physician's lack of concrete criteria and the theologian's dogmatism, it can be argued that there is a middle course that entails substantive criteria to assist decision-makers regarding treatment decisions for handicapped newborns. McCormick has proposed a patient-centered, quality-of-life criterion that can be used by appropriate decision-makers in determining treatment decisions for handicapped newborns. The significance of McCormick's quality-of-life criterion is that it offers the appropriate decision-makers, for never-competent newborns, a practical, beneficial, and appropriate moral criterion that is not only reasonable and coherent but is grounded in a tradition that promotes the best interests of handicapped newborns.

The purpose of this article is threefold: first, to present a case of a child born with thanatophoric dysplasia; second to examine McCormick's moral criterion as it applies to the anomaly presented and to five diagnostic treatment categories, established by this author, which span the spectrum of neonatal defects; third, to assess whether McCormick's moral criterion is an appropriate moral criterion for the decision-makers of handicapped newborns.

2. Case study – Thanatophoric dysplasia

On September 25, 2004 Baby X was born with a genetic condition called thanatophoric dysplasia. His condition was diagnosed in utero and upon birth he was placed on mechanical ventilation to give the medical team additional time to confirm the diagnosis. Besides mechanical ventilation the child also received artificial nutrition and hydration through a feeding tube and was kept unconscious and sedated for comfort. After numerous consultations from various pediatric specialists the medical team decided that to continue aggressive medical treatment was futile and only prolonged the child's dying process. The child's mother was unsure if withholding aggressive medical treatment was ethical and sought additional guidance.

Thanatophoric dysplasia (TD), also called thanatophoric dwarfism, was discovered in 1967 by Pierre Maroteaux and his coworkers who used the Greek term "thanatophoric" meaning death-bringing. It is the most common form of skeletal dysplasia in humans. It occurs in 3 to 4 per 100,000 live births and is due to autosomal dominant sporadic *de novo* mutations in the fibroblast growth factor receptor 3 (FGFR3) gene mapped to chromosome band 4p16.3. This gene codes for the FGFR3 transmembrane receptor expressed largely by skeletal and brain tissues in the developing fetus where it is involved with growth regulation.[7] Male and female fetuses are equally affected. There are two subtypes, TD1 and TD2, based on genetic-phenotypic differences, although features may overlap. TD1 is associated with radiographic findings of short curved ("telephone receiver") femurs, with or without a clover-leaf skull deformity. TD2 is associated with straight, longer femurs, and clover-leaf skull. The genetic mutation responsible for TD1 leads to an arginine to cysteine amino acid substitution at position 248, whereas for TD2, it leads to a lysine to glutamine substitution at position 650 of the FGFR3 receptor.[8] However, the distinction does not alter the management.

Neonates with TD invariably develop severe respiratory distress at birth due to lung hypoplasia requiring ventilation. The only means available to treat this condition is respiratory support. If the diagnosis is known ante-natally, then the parents would have the option of withholding active resuscitation. However, if the diagnosis is uncertain then, active resuscitation will buy time for further investigations until the diagnosis is determined. Physical findings manifest at birth include a bulging forehead, proptosis, flat nasal bridge, narrow chest, protuberant abdomen, and short limbs. A babygram should be done which may reveal characteristic telephone receiver femurs, flaring of the long bone metaphyses, short ribs, flat vertebral bodies, widened intervertebral disk spaces, a short pelvis with small sacroiliac notch, and cloverleaf skull deformity.[9]

Most babies with TD die within the first few hours of life from respiratory insufficiency secondary to reduced thoracic capacity or compression of the brainstem. Management concerns are limited to extreme life support measures for the newborn. In the rare cases of long-term survival (a 4.7 year male and 3.7 year female),[10] the management consists in treatment of manifestations: respiratory support (tracheostomy, ventilation); medication to control seizures; shunt placement when hydrocephaly is identified; suboccipital decompression for relief of craniocervical junction constriction; hearing aids when hearing loss is identified and orthopedic evaluation upon development of joint contractures of joint hypermobility.[11]

This case is an excellent example of how parents in consultation with health care professionals struggle to decide whether certain medical treatments are medically proportionate or disproportionate and in the best interest of the child.

3. McCormick's criterion

McCormick will determine how treatment decisions are made for handicapped newborns by proposing his normative understanding of best interests which evolves gradually into his quality-of-life criterion. This is a patient-centered, teleological assessment, which is based on a normative understanding of what reasonable persons ought to choose in a particular situation for the never-competent patient.[12] It appears that McCormick's quality-of-life criterion is nothing more than a further specification of his normative understanding of best interests.[13] McCormick has a normative understanding of best interests because, as social beings, our good, our flourishing (therefore, our best interests) is inextricably bound up with the well-being of others".[14] The best interests category is a composite category that involves quality-of-life considerations, benefit-burden considerations, and the use of proportionate reason as a tool for establishing what is promotive or destructive for the good of the person integrally and adequately considered".[15] McCormick understands quality of life to be an elusive term whose meaning varies according to context. However, at a more profound level, when the issue is preserving human life, the term assumes a more basic meaning. "Just as life itself is a condition for any other value or achievement, so certain characteristics of life are the conditions for the achievement of other values. We must distinguish between two sets of conditions: those that allow us to do things well, easily, comfortably, and efficiently, and those that allow us to do them at all".[16] The quality-of-life criterion is ethically significant for parents and health care professionals, because it represents not only the value of the whole person, but it affirms that respect for the human person entails considering all the relevant factors and circumstances that are involved in any situation.

There are real difficulties in trying to establish a perfectly rational criterion for making quality-of-life judgments. To make his quality-of-life criterion more concrete, McCormick will establish two guidelines and four norms that will further specify his criterion. The first guideline developed for dealing with never-competent patients focuses on the potential for human relationships associated with the infant's condition. By relational potential McCormick means "the hope that the infant will, in relative comfort, be able to experience our caring and love".[17] Specifically, he proposes that "if a newborn baby had no potential for such relationships or if the potential would be totally submerged in the mere struggle to survive, then that baby had achieved its potential and further life-prolonging efforts were not mandatory, that is, would no longer be in the best interests of the baby".[18] Therefore, according to this guideline, when a never-competent patient, even with treatment, will have no potential for human relationships, the appropriate decision-makers can decide to withhold treatment and allow the patient to die.[19] McCormick claims this quality-of-life approach has its foundation in the traditional ordinary-extraordinary means distinction that was later clarified by Pius XII.[20] This is not an easy guideline to apply, especially in the case of never-competent patients. In essence, this guideline requires that the appropriate decision-makers must be able to determine if a minimally accepted quality of life can be expected. This determination ought to be made on the basis of the never-competent's best interests understood normatively. This guideline does not depreciate the value of the never-competent individual but affirms that a genuine respect for the person demands attention to the prospects held out by continued life.[21]

This guideline of the potential for human relationships has been criticized for being too general and open to possible abuse.[22] McCormick himself stated when he advanced this guideline that it was "general and rather vague. But this is the way it is with all moral norms." [23] Despite being convinced that this guideline is fundamentally sound, McCormick understood that he must further concretize it. Specifically, there are those circumstances when the never-competent patient has the potential for human relationships, but the underlying medical condition is critical and will result in imminent death, or after treatment has been initiated it becomes apparent that the treatment is medically futile.[24] In these two situations it is clear that, besides the potential for human relationships, McCormick must incorporate an additional guideline that can weigh the benefits and burdens of certain treatments.

The second guideline of McCormick=s quality-of-life criterion is the benefit-burden evaluation. "Where medical procedures are in question, it is generally admitted that the criterion to be used is a benefits-burdens estimate . . . The question posed is: Will the burden of the treatment outweigh the benefits to the patient? The general answer: If the treatment is useless or futile, or it imposes burdens that outweigh the benefits, it may be omitted".[25] As is the case with his first guideline, McCormick claims the benefit-burden evaluation emerges out of the ordinary-extraordinary means distinction.

McCormick believes that his notion of benefit-burden evaluation within his quality-of-life criterion is a logical development of the ordinary-extraordinary means distinction, or what he refers to as an extension of the tradition into new problem areas.[26] McCormick believes that the ordinary-extraordinary means distinction has an honorable history and an enduring validity. However, he argues that these terms "summarize and promulgate judgments drawn on other grounds. It is these other grounds that cry out for explication".[27] To further explain these other grounds, McCormick reformulates the ordinary-extraordinary means distinction by advancing his benefit-burden evaluation. An extraordinary means is one that offers the patient no real benefit, or offers it at a disproportionate cost. For McCormick, one is called to make a moral judgment: Does the benefit of a proposed medical intervention really outweigh the harm it will inevitably produce? This is a quality-of-life judgment. The benefit-burden interpretation is not a departure from the Catholic tradition. It is a reformulation of the tradition in order to deal with contemporary bioethical problem areas.[28]

The reason for this reformulation of the tradition is that over the centuries the ordinary-extraordinary means distinction has become less objective and more relative because medicine and technology have become more sophisticated. The medical profession is committed to curing disease and preserving life. Today, we have the medical technology to make this commitment a reality. However, McCormick argues that "this commitment must be implemented within a healthy and realistic acknowledgment that we are mortal."[29] Therefore, there is a need to reformulate the basic value of human life under new circumstances. For many contemporary ethicists the traditional terminology of ordinary-extraordinary means has outlived its usefulness and could take us only so far, especially in the case of handicapped newborns.[30] Focusing on the value of human life, McCormick sought to reformulate the ordinary-extraordinary means distinction without abandoning the tradition. Contemporary medical problems no longer only concern newborns for whom biological death is imminent. Modern medicine and technology have the ability to keep almost anyone biologically alive. Therefore, a gradual shift has occurred from the means to reverse the dying process to the quality of life sustained and preserved as the result of the application of medical technology.[31] Today, because of the advancements in medicine and technology, the focus is on the quality of life thus saved that establishes a means as extraordinary.

To address this shift in the problem from means to quality of life preserved, McCormick has reformulated the ordinary-extraordinary means distinction to mean the benefit-burden evaluation.[32] For McCormick, "it is clear that the judgments of burden and benefit are value judgments, moral choices. They are judgments in which, all things considered, the continuance of life is either called for or not worthwhile to the patient."[33] In making these moral judgments one can see how proportionate reason is used as a tool for determining whether a particular life-sustaining treatment is a benefit or a burden, that is, in the best interests of the never-competent patient and those involved in the decision-making process.

The benefit-burden evaluation was also proposed by the Sacred Congregation for the Doctrine of the Faith in its *Declaration on Euthanasia* and by the President's Commission for the Study of Ethical Problems in Medicine and Biomedical and Behavioral Research in its *Deciding to Forego Life-Sustaining Treatment*.[34] The issuance of the *Declaration on Euthanasia* in 1980 by the Magisterium gave McCormick further justification for incorporating the benefit-burden evaluation into his quality-of-life criterion.[35] It also gave him further proof to anchor his guideline and thus his criterion for treatment decisions in the benefit-burden evaluation. Medical treatments are not morally mandatory if they are either gravely burdensome or useless for the patient.[36] McCormick has a normative understanding of medical futility, which considers whether the agreed on potential effect is of any value and benefit to the newborn, that is, in the newborn's best interests normatively understood. For McCormick, a medical treatment might be successful in achieving an effect (physiologically effective), but the effect might not be beneficial to the patient (qualitatively effective). Since the goal of medical treatment is to benefit the patient, it follows that nonbeneficial treatment is medically futile.[37] This entails making a value judgment and the evaluation of whether a treatment is a benefit or a burden can be open to personal interpretation. That means these evaluations can be borderline and controversial.[38]

The two guidelines of McCormick's quality-of-life criterion, even though he argued they were both reformulations of the ordinary-extraordinary means distinction, continued to be criticized by ethicists Leonard Weber, John Connery and Warren Reich for being too relative, subjective, and consequential in nature. To address this criticism McCormick, along with ethicist John Paris, S.J., proposed the following norms that would further specify the capacity for human relationships and the benefit-burden evaluation:

1. Life-saving intervention ought not to be omitted for institutional or managerial reasons. Included in this specification is the ability of this particular family to cope with a badly disabled baby.
2. Life-sustaining interventions may not be omitted simply because the baby is retarded. There may be further complications associated with retardation that justify withholding life-sustaining treatment.
3. Life-sustaining intervention may be omitted or withdrawn when there is excessive hardship on the patient, especially when this combines with poor prognosis.
4. Life-sustaining interventions may be omitted or withdrawn at a point when it becomes clear that expected life can be had only for a relatively brief time and only with continued use of artificial feeding.[39]

These norms or rules do not mandate certain decisions, nor do they replace the role of prudence and eliminate conflicts and decisions. They are simply attempts to provide outlines of the areas in which prudence should operate.[40]

McCormick further specified his quality-of-life criterion to help enlighten medical situations for the appropriate decision-makers. However, guidelines, even specified by concrete norms, cannot cover all circumstances and every possible situation. McCormick's quality-of-life criterion assists the appropriate decision-makers by giving them a range of choices. As rational persons, it is up to the appropriate decision-makers to examine each situation using proportionate reason, and the guidelines advanced by McCormick in his quality-of-life criterion, to determine what is in the best interests of the never-competent patient and those involved in the decision-making process. McCormick makes clear that no criterion can cover every instance where human discretion must intervene to decide. There is always the possibility of human error because we are finite and sinful people. For McCormick, "the margin of error tolerable should reflect not only the utter finality of the decision (which tends to narrow it), but also the unavoidable uncertainty and doubt (which tends to broaden it)".[41] With the assistance of these guidelines and norms, McCormick believes that the appropriate decision-makers will be given the necessary guidance to act responsibly.

To assist parents and health care professionals further in medical decision-making for handicapped newborns five specific diagnostic treatment categories of handicapped newborns have been established. These categories attempt to encompass, as far as possible, the entire spectrum of handicapped newborns. They are based on McCormick's moral criterion of the potential for human relationships.

McCormick has plotted the two extreme positions on this spectrum of handicapped newborns, but has left the conflictual middle, to be filled in by health care professionals and bioethicsts.[42] These diagnostic categories will attempt to complete the conflictual middle. The conflictual middle pertains to those neonatal anomalies that fall into the gray area of treatment decisions.[43] These diagnostic treatment categories have been arranged in a way that demonstrates the application of McCormick's best interests category. There is a logical progression on the spectrum from the newborn who does not warrant medical treatment to the newborn who does warrant medical treatment. The five diagnostic treatment categories are:

1. The handicapped newborns whose potential for human relationships is completely nonexistent.
2. The handicapped newborn who has a potential for human relationships but whose potential is utterly submerged in the mere struggle for survival.
3. The handicapped newborn who has a potential for human relationships but the underlying medical condition will result in imminent death.
4. The handicapped newborn who has the potential for human relationships but after medical treatment has been initiated, it becomes apparent that the treatment may be medically futile.
5. The handicapped newborn who has the potential for human relationships and has a correctable or treatable condition.[44]

Establishing a full set of diagnostic treatment categories is not a panacea for determining treatment decisions for handicapped newborns. Not all medical conditions can be placed in specific categories; there is a marked difference in the severity of conditions within each category. Not all health care professionals or even bioethicists could or would agree to these specific categories. Nevertheless, as McCormick argues, "we ought to attempt, as far as possible, to approach neonatal disabilities through diagnostic categories, always realizing that such categories cannot deflate important differences and that there will always remain gray areas."[45] The establishment of these five diagnostic treatment categories is an attempt to meet the challenge set before health care professionals and bioethicists to assist parents and medical professionals in making treatment decisions for handicapped newborns.

4. Ethical evaluation

In the case of Baby X, the medical professionals have ascertained after five months that any further aggressive medical treatment would be medically futile for this child. According to the physicians, Baby X has severe underdeveloped lungs, ribs too tiny to allow normal breathing and pressure on the spinal cord that disrupts brain signals controlling respiration. Thus, Baby X is in a terminal condition and is slowly suffocating. Mechanical ventilation at this point is only prolonging the dying process. It would appear that Baby X would fit under diagnostic category four.

In this fourth diagnostic treatment category, since the potential for human relationships is present, McCormick's second guideline of his quality-of-life criterion--the benefit-burden evaluation--would be applied to determine whether Baby X ought to be treated. What is to be determined is whether the benefit of the treatment will outweigh the burden to the newborn. If the parents in consultation with the health care professionals determine that further medical treatment would not improve the newborn=s prognosis, or benefit the overall well-being of the newborn, then, all things considered, parents should decide that further treatment would not be in the best interests of the newborn. A newborn diagnosed with thanatophoric dysplasia is in a terminal condition and according to medical authorities, further medical treatment is medically futile, that is, any possible medical effect is of no benefit to the newborn. To support this position McCormick's third norm, that further specifies the burden-benefit evaluation, can be applied. "Life sustaining interventions may be omitted or withdrawn when there is excessive hardship, especially when this combines with poor prognosis." Therefore, it appears that further treatment for Baby X is not morally obligatory, because it is a disproportionate means.

The notion of a normative understanding of best interests considers not only the relevant medical facts but also the relevant social and familial factors. Financial and emotional costs ought to be considered. That means, if the social factors are excessive, then the newborn should not and would not want to be treated, because it would place excessive burdens on those who must care for the newborn's existence. What the newborn ought to want should encompass the needs of those who will care for this child. Baby X is in a terminal state and further aggressive treatments will only prolong the dying process. Both social and familial factors ought to play a proportionate role in determining the benefit/burden evaluation.[46]

In conclusion, when a handicapped newborn has the potential for human relationships but after initiating treatment, it becomes apparent that the treatment is medically futile, parents in consultation with health care professionals are not morally obliged to continue medical treatment. This is a value judgment that is based on McCormick's guidelines of relational potential and benefit/burden evaluation. McCormick's moral criterion sets basic parameters and enlightens the particular medical situation. Ultimately, the parents will use prudence to examine the medical facts and to weigh, all things considered, whether the burdens of treatment outweigh the benefits to the newborn. In this diagnostic treatment category, the burdens and benefits need to be weighed carefully. However, with the severity of this particular medical anomaly the burdens clearly outweigh the benefits to the newborn. Therefore, in the best interests of the newborn, and all concerned, parents in consultation with health care professionals have the moral obligation to forgo or withdraw treatment for a newborn in these circumstances.

McCormick argues that his moral criterion is appropriate for decision-makers because it considers not only the relevant medical facts and the pertinent circumstances of the situation, but also familial and social factors, such as, religious, cultural, emotional, and financial factors. Parents in consultation with health care professionals can best determine what the handicapped newborn ought to want and protect his or her best interests by using McCormick's quality-of-life moral criterion. As reasonable people, parents are most knowledgeable about the family situation into which the newborn is born. This includes knowing the financial, emotional, and social factors. Parents can also weigh and balance the religious and cultural values that inform their decision-making. Health care professionals have the specialized medical knowledge and clinical expertise that can assist parents in the decision-making process. They also have a level of objectivity that parents may lack because of the overwhelming emotional stress of the situation. Together, parents and health care professionals are able to determine what are the appropriate needs of this newborn, to assess these needs, and to determine whether medical treatment is in the best interests of the newborn integrally and adequately considered.

5. Conclusion

McCormick's moral criterion is appropriate for Christian decision-makers because it emphasizes the reasonable from within a Christian context. It stresses the need for decision-makers to examine the medical facts, the circumstances of the situation, foreseeable consequences, social and familial factors, and other pertinent data before deciding on an appropriate course of action. McCormick's moral criterion also stresses that these facts are to be considered always within the context of the Christian story, so that the best interests of the handicapped newborn are always promoted and protected. Treatment decisions for handicapped newborns are value judgments that must be based on the appropriate needs of the newborn. These value judgments can possibly become distorted by self-interested perspectives and technological considerations. Christian decision-makers who use McCormick's moral criterion are not immune from making mistakes. We are a finite and sinful people. What is being said is that because the content of this moral criterion is reasonable, and because these decisions are made within the context of the Christian story, less chance exists that such treatment decisions will be pushed to the extremes. McCormick's moral criterion is appropriate for Christian decision-makers because it protects the best interests of the handicapped newborns by promoting value judgments that are grounded in reason and informed by the Christian story.

6. References

[1] For a more detailed analysis of the 1984 Child Abuse Law, see Department of Health and Human Services, AChild Abuse and Neglect: Prevention and Treatment,@ reprinted from The Federal Register 50 (April 15, 1985), no. 72: Rules and Regulations, part 1340, 14887-14892.

[2] For a more detailed analysis of the guidelines of the American Academy of Pediatrics, see American Academy of Pediatrics, AJoint Policy Statement: Principles Of Treatment Of Disabled Infants,@ Pediatrics 73 (1984): 559-560; and American Academy of Pediatrics, AGuidelines For Infant Bioethics Review Committees,@ Pediatrics 74 (1984): 306-310.

[3] There is an ethical distinction regarding competent, noncompetent and never-competent patients. A competent patient is one who can make decisions regarding health care for him or herself. A noncompetent patient is one who was once competent, but now lacks that decision-making capacity. A never-competent patient is one who never had this decision-making capacity and never will have it in the future.

[4] James Castelli, ARichard A. McCormick, S.J., And Life/Death Decisions,@ St. Anthony Messenger 83 (August 1975): 34. McCormick, as interviewed by Castelli.

[5] McCormick uses as an example the traditional obligation to preserve life. He argues that the Christian tradition Ahas always strived to maintain a middle course between two extremes: medical-moral utopianism, i.e., sustaining life at all costs and with

all means because when life is over everything is over and death is an absolute end, and its opposite, medical-moral pessimism, i.e., there is no point in sustaining life if it is accompanied by suffering, lack of function, etc. Both of these extremes are basic devaluations of human life because they remove life from the context which gives it its ultimate significance. The middle path is a recognition of the facts that human life is a basic value, the most basic value, because it is the foundation for all other values and achievements, but that life is not the absolute good and death the ultimate and absolute evil.@ McCormick, AA Proposal For >Quality Of Life= Criteria For Sustaining Life,@ Hospital Progress 56 (September 1975): 76.

[6] Richard A. McCormick, ATo Save Or Let Die,@ How Brave A New World?: Dilemmas In Bioethics, (Garden City, N.Y.: Doubleday, 1981), 342.

[7] D. W. Bianchi, T.M. Crombleholme, M.E. D'Alton ME, "Thanatophoric Dysplasia," in D.W. Bianchi, T.M. Crombleholme, M.E. D'Alton, editors *Fetology: Diagnosis and Management of the Fetal Patient* (New York: McGraw-Hill, 2000): 751-759.

[8] Ibid.

[9] Ibid.

[10] I.M McDonald, A.G. Hunter, P.M. MacLeod et al., "Growth and Development in Thanatophoric Dysplasia," *American Journal of Medical Genetics* 33 (1989): 508-512.

[11] Elio Liboi, Patricia Lievens, "Thanatophoric Dysplasia," *Orphanet Encyclopedia*, September 2004, 1-6.
http://www.prpha.net/data/patho/GB/uk-Thanatophoric-dysplasia.pdf

[12] The structure and individual components that makeup McCormick=s moral criterion for decision-making are normative; they center on what Aought@ to be the case, not what Ais@ the case. By normative McCormick means what the never-competent patient would want because he or she Aought@ to want it. The never-competent patient Aought@ to make this choice because it is in his/her Abest interests.@ For a more detailed analysis of McCormick=s position on a normative understanding of his patient-centered approach, see McCormick, AThe Rights Of The Voiceless,@ How Brave A New World?, 99-113.

[13] Ethicist Robert Weir disagrees with McCormick on this point. Weir argues that the quality-of-life criterion and best interests criterion are distinct and separate. McCormick responds to Weir by stating: AI believe Weir is wrong when he asserts that for those who use quality-of-life assessment, >it is not necessary to consider the best interest of the neonate.= It is precisely because one is focused on best interests that qualitative considerations cannot be ignored but indeed are central. Weir is clearly afraid that quality-of-life considerations will be unfair. But they need not be. It all depends on where the line is drawn. I am all the more convinced of the inseparable unity and general overlap of best interests and quality-of-life considerations when I study Weir=s clinical applications of his ethical criteria.@ McCormick, review of Selective Nontreatment Of Handicapped Newborns, by Robert Weir, in Perspectives In Biology And Medicine 29 (Winter 1986): 328.

[14] McCormick, AThe Rights Of The Voiceless,@ How Brave A New World?, 101. It should be noted that McCormick=s understanding of Abest interests@ is grounded in his Arevised@ natural law position. AI believe we do have reasons for assuming we know in many cases what an incompetent would want. We may assume that most people are reasonable, and that being such they would choose what is in their best interest. At least this is a safe and protective guideline to follow in structuring our conduct toward them when they cannot speak. The assumption may be factually and *per accidens* incorrect. But I am convinced that it will not often be. . . . I believe

most of us want to act reasonably within parameters that are objective in character, even though we do not always do so. Or at least I think it good protective policy to assume this.@ Ibid., 104-105.

[15] It should be noted that when McCormick refers to benefits in his Abest interests@ category it is not restricted to medical benefits. Benefits also apply to social and familial benefits. This notion of Abenefit@ originates in Pellegrino=s four components of Abest interests@ that McCormick has incorporated into his Abest interests@ category. For a more detailed analysis of Pellegrino=s position, see Edmund Pellegrino, M.D., AMoral Choice, The Good Of The Patient And The Patient=s Good,@ in Ethics And Critical Care Medicine, eds. J. C. Moskop & L. Kopelman (Dordrecht, Netherlands: D. Reidel, 1985), 117-138.

[16] McCormick, AA Proposal For AQuality Of Life@ Criteria For Sustaining Life,@ 77-78.

[17] McCormick, ATo Save Or Let Die,@ 351.

[18] McCormick, AThe Best Interests Of The Baby,@ Second Opinion 2 (1986): 23.

[19] This does not mean that once a decision has been made to forego or discontinue treatment, that the dying person is not treated with dignity and respect. For McCormick, even though a person has reached his or her potential and no treatment is recommended, as members of society we still have a moral obligation to give comfort to the person while he or she is in the dying process. That comfort would consist in palliative care. Palliative care is aimed at controlling pain, relieving discomfort, and aiding dysfunction of various sorts.

[20] McCormick quotes Pius XII as saying that an obligation to use any means possible Awould be too burdensome for most men and would render the attainment of the higher, more important good too difficult.@ Pius XII, AThe Prolongation Of Life,@ *Acta Apostolicae Sedis* 49 (1957): 1,031-1,032. McCormick understands Pius XII to say that certain treatments may be refused because it would lead to a life that lacks the proper quality. Leonard J. Weber, Who Shall Live?: The Dilemma Of Severely Handicapped Children And Its Meaning For Other Moral Questions, (New York: Paulist Press, 1976), 69.

[21] Lisa Sowle Cahill, AOn Richard McCormick: Reason And Faith In Post-Vatican II Catholic Ethics,,@ in Theological Voices In Medical Ethics eds. Allen Verhey & Stephen Lammers (Grand Rapids, MI.: William B. Eerdmans Publishing Co., 1993): 91. The potential for human relationships is based in the Catholic tradition. McCormick bases this potential for human relationships in the Catholic tradition. The Christian story does not yield concrete answers and fixed rules, but it does yield various perspectives and insights that inform human reasoning. One such insight is that human life is a basic good but not an absolute good. Since human life is a relative good, and the duty to preserve it is a limited one, then it is not always morally obligatory to use all means to preserve human life if a person cannot attain the higher more important good. For McCormick, the Ahigher@ more important good is the capacity for relationships of love. The core of this guideline is developed from the love commandment found in the New Testament.

[22] Both Leonard Weber and John Connery have criticized McCormick=s quality-of-life criterion. For a more detailed analysis, see Weber, Who Shall Live?: The Dilemma Of Severely Handicapped Children And Its Meaning For Other Moral Questions (New York: Paulist Press, 1976) and John Connery, AQuality Of Life,@ Linacre Quarterly 53 (February 1986): 26-33.

[23] AThey really root in general assertions that must be fleshed out by experience, modified by discussion and consultation, propped up and strengthened by

cautions and qualifications. It is in the process of their application that moral norms take on added concreteness.@McCormick, ATo Save Or Let Die: State Of The Questions,@ America 131 (October 5, 1974): 171.

[24] It should be noted that the term Amedically futile@ is an elusive and ambiguous term. There are four major types of medical futility. First, physiological futility--an intervention cannot lead to the intended physiological effect. Second, imminent demise futility--an intervention may be futile if despite that intervention the patient will die in the very near future (this is sometimes expressed as the patient will not survive to discharge, although that is not really equivalent to dying in the near future). Third, lethal condition futility--an intervention may be futile if the patient has an underlying lethal condition which the intervention does not affect and which will result in death in the not too far future (weeks, perhaps months, but not in years) even if the intervention is employed. Fourth, qualitative futility--an intervention may be futile if it fails to lead to an acceptable quality of life. For a more detailed analysis of medical futility, see Baruch A. Brody and Amir Halevy, AIs Futility A Futile Concept?@ Journal Of Medicine And Philosophy 20 (April 1995): 126-129.

[25] Richard A. McCormick, S.J., ATechnology And Morality: The Example Of Medicine,@ New Theology Review 2 (November 1989): 26.

[26] McCormick writes: AA basic human value is challenged by new circumstances, and these circumstances demand that imagination and creativity be employed to devise new formulations, a new understanding of this value in light of these new circumstances while retaining a basic grasp upon the value. For example, in-vitro fertilization poses questions about the meaning of sexuality, parenthood, and the family because it challenges their very biological roots.@ McCormick, AA Proposal For >Quality Of Life= Criteria For Sustaining Life,@ 76.

[27] McCormick, AThe Best Interests Of The Baby,@ 19. McCormick further states: AWe must admit that the terms >ordinary= and >extraordinary= are but code words. That is, they summarize and are vehicles for other judgments. They do not solve problems automatically. Rather they are emotional and mental preparations for very personal and circumstantial judgments that must take into account the patient=s attitudes and value perspectives, or >what the patient would have wanted.= >Ordinary= and >extraordinary= merely summarize other underlying judgments. They say very little in and of themselves.@ McCormick, AA Proposal For >Quality Of Life= Criteria For Sustaining Life,@ 77.

[28] McCormick further states that: AIt must be remembered that the abiding substance of the Church=s teaching, its rock bottom so to speak, is not found in the ordinary means-extraordinary means terminology. It is found in a basic value judgment about the meaning of life and death, one that refuses to absolutize either. It is *that judgment* that we must carry with us as we face the medical decisions that technology casts upon us.@ McCormick, ATechnology And Morality: An Example Of Medicine,@ 29. Emphasis in the original.

[29] Richard McCormick, The Critical Calling: Moral Dilemmas Since Vatican II (Washington, D.C.: Georgetown University Press, 1989), 365.

[30] McCormick argues there are two reasons for this: First, the terminology too easily hides the nature of the judgment being made. The major reference point in factoring out what is Areasonable@ (benefit) and Aexcessive@ (burden) is the patient--his or her condition, biography, prognosis, and values. The terminology, however, suggests that attention should fall on the means in an all too mechanical way. Second, many people misinterpret the terms to refer to Awhat physicians

ordinarily do, what is customary.@ This is not what the term means. In their ethical sense, they encompass many more dimensions of the situation. Richard McCormick, Health And Medicine In The Catholic Tradition, (New York: Crossroad Press, 1987), 145.

[31] McCormick, ATo Save Or Let Die,@ How Brave A New World?, 345.

[32] Besides McCormick=s benefit-burden evaluation, other ethicists have suggested various terms to reformulate the ordinary-extraordinary means distinction. Paul Ramsey suggests that the morally significant meaning of ordinary and extraordinary medical means can be reduced almost without remainder to two components--a comparison of treatments to determine if they are Amedically indicated@ and a patient=s right to refuse treatment. See Paul Ramsey, Ethics At The Edges Of Life: Moral And Legal Intersections, (New Haven, CT.: Yale University Press, 1978), 153-160. Robert Veatch maintains that the terms Aordinary@ and Aextraordinary@ are Aextremely vague and are used inconsistently in the literature.@ Beneath this confusion he finds three overlapping but fundamentally different uses of the terms: usual versus unusual, useful versus useless, imperative versus elective. See Robert Veatch, Death, Dying And The Biological Revolution, (New Haven, CT.: Yale University Press, 1976), 110-112. For further examples, see McCormick, AThe Quality Of Life, The Sanctity Of Life,@ How Brave A New World?, 393-405.

[33] McCormick and John Paris, ASaving Defective Infants,@ How Brave A New World?, 360.

[34] See President=s Commission For The Study Of Ethical Problems In Medicine And Biomedical And Behavioral Research, ADeciding To Forego Life-Sustaining Treatment: Ethical, Medical And Legal Issues In Treatment Decisions,@ (Washington, D.C., U.S. Printing Office, March 1983): 218-219.

[35] The Congregation concludes that, Ait will be possible to make a correct judgment as to the means by studying the type of treatment being used, its degree of complexity or risk, its cost and possibilities of using it, and comparing these elements with the result that can be expected, taking into account the state of the sick person and his or her physical and moral resources.@ Congregation for the Doctrine of the Faith, ADeclaration On Euthanasia,@ Origins 10 (August 1980): 263.

[36] Ethicists Warren Reich, John Connery, S.J., Leonard Weber, and Donald McCarthy disagree with McCormick=s interpretation of the tradition on the benefit-burden distinction. Ethicist Richard Sparks writes: AFor Reich, Weber, Connery, and McCarthy the limiting factor is the quality of life, which, if judged to be excessively burdensome, can make the presumably beneficial treatment extraordinary and optional, [sic] must be caused by or directly related to the use of the means contemplated. In other words, >the burden must be the burden of medical treatment, not the burden of handicapped existence.=@ Richard Sparks, To Treat Or Not To Treat?: Bioethics And The Handicapped Newborn, (New York: Paulist Press, 1988), 110; see also Donald G. McCarthy, ATreating Defective Newborns: Who Judges Extraordinary Means?@ Hospital Progress 62 (December 1981): 45-50; John Connery, S.J., AProlongation Of Life: A Duty And Its Limits,@ Linacre Quarterly 47 (May 1980):, 151-165; Leonard Weber, Who Shall Live?, 88-98; and Warren Reich, AQuality Of Life And Defective Newborn Children: An Ethical Analysis,@ in Decision-Making And The Defective Newborn, ed. Chester A. Swinyard (Springfield, IL.: Thomas, 1978), 488 -511.

[37] For McCormick, medical futility is determined by the parents in consultation with the health care professionals, because a determination must be made of the patient=s medical status and an evaluation must be made of the medical intervention. The determination of medical futility entails balancing the values of patients, the values of medicine, and the fact that there is much uncertainty in making Apredictive medical judgments.@ McCormick=s notion of medical futility is also rooted in his understanding of the principles of beneficence and nonmaleficence--do no harm to the patient. For a more detailed analysis of medical futility, see James F. Drane and John L. Coulehan, AThe Concept Of Futility: Parents Do Not Have The Right To Demand Medically Useless Treatment,@ Health Progress 74 (December 1993): 32; Robert Veatch and Carol Mason Spicer, AFutile Care: Physicians Should Not Be Allowed To Refuse To Treat,@ Health Progress 74 (December 1993): 22-27 and Glenn G. Griener, AThe Physician=s Authority To Withhold Futile Treatment,@ Journal Of Philosophy And Medicine 20 (April 1995): 209..

[38] McCormick and Paris, ASaving Defective Infants,@ How Brave A New World?, 358.

[39] Ibid., 358-359.

[40] Ibid., 359.

[41] Ibid., 360.

[42] McCormick writes: AIt is the task of physicians to provide some more concrete categories or presumptive biological symptoms for this human judgment. For instance, nearly all would likely agree that the anencephalic infant is without relational potential. On the other hand, the same cannot be said for the mongoloid infant. The task ahead is to attach relational potential to presumptive biological symptoms for the gray areas between such extremes.@ McCormick, ATo Save Or Let Die,@ How Brave_A New World?, 349-350.

[43] This would include anomalies in which the newborn has the potential for human relationships, but the potential is utterly submerged in the mere struggle for survival, or the medical condition will result in imminent death, or it has been determined that further treatment is medically futile. Certain anomalies that would fall within this category would be spina bifida, hypoplastic left heart syndrome, trisomy 13, trisomy 18, Lesch-Nyhan syndrome, etc.

[44] For a more complete analysis of these five diagnostic categories see, Peter A. Clark, *To Treat Or Not To Treat: The Ethical Methodology of Richard A. McCormick, S.J. As Applied To Treatment Decisions For Handicapped Newborns*, (Omaha, Ne.: Creighton University Press, 2003).

[45] McCormick, AThe Best Interests Of The Baby,@ 24.

[46] It should be noted that McCormick=s position on social and familial factors has been criticized for being too restrictive and deviating from both the Catholic tradition and from his own normative understanding of Abest interests.@ McCormick claims that his restrictive notion of social and familial factors, as they pertain to treatment decisions for handicapped newborns, is due to the fact that a broader interpretation could lead to social utilitarianism. This caution is certainly relevant because the possibility of potential abuse is always present. However, the safeguards McCormick has built into his quality-of-life criterion--guidelines and norms--should help to alleviate the possibility of such abuse. In addition, health care professionals serve as a safeguard in that they can act as the newborn=s advocate should they suspect abuse.

6

Ethics in Pharmaceutical Issues

M. I. Noordin
Department of Pharmacy,
Faculty of Medicine,
University of Malaya,
Malaysia

1. Introduction

Pharmacists are the researchers, developers, producers, people who are trusted to give advice on drugs to all health professionals and persons who market drugs in the whole world. The pharmaceutical industry is the most heavily regulated of all industries. Clearly we can say that this profession and this industry is the most heavily reliant on a code of ethics in its everyday practice.

A music writer is a professional in his own personal way; another professional, a musician, can play his music but he cannot write in the way that the writer did. In a similar manner, a doctor knows how to use a medicine but he cannot produce the medicine. This task is undertaken by another professional, the pharmacist. Pharmacists dispense prescription drug products and provide patient information services to consumers in hospitals, nursing homes, retail pharmacy departments and home care settings. Pharmacists consult directly with patients, or with their caregivers, explaining the proper use and storage of drug products and providing information on contraindications of drugs.

Generally, dictionaries define ethics as the issues related to the general nature of morals and of the specific moral choices to be made by a person. In other words, ethics are derived from the moral philosophy of a person. Personal philosophy makes a significant part of any discussion of ethics. Ethics can be influenced by one's family values, educational background, social learning, professional activities, religious beliefs, and individual needs. For a pharmacist, professionalism is the main driving force for ethical conduct. There may not be a common global standard on the code of ethics of pharmacists but every nation will have a set of guidelines on the code of ethics or code of conduct for pharmacists. Each country's pharmacy professional body, board or council will use the code of ethics or code of conduct to safeguard the profession. Such a code of ethics or code of conduct will be used as a guide by the professional body on action to be taken for misconduct or infamous conduct of the member pharmacists.

It is globally known that the national Board of Registration of Pharmacists or similar bodies provides a code of professional conduct to ensure the highest degree of ethical and moral practice by pharmacists. These bodies will also monitor pharmacists to ensure they meet the standard of ethics as stipulated. The pharmacist code of ethics is to ensure that consumers are receiving the highest quality drug products with assured safety and efficacy. Furthermore the national Board of Registration of Pharmacists or similar bodies will also usually set standards for the curriculum of pharmacy in their country. There will be a check list on the content of the curriculum, where will include a requirement on the teaching of ethics as a formal course.

2. Pharmacy historical role

Briefly we can learn about the historical role of a pharmacist or a pharmacy by going back into history, from the era of the Greeks and the Romans, the influence of the Muslim Caliphate, the era of the crusaders and the era of the industrial revolution in Europe and the establishment of a new nation, the United States of America.

The art of pharmacy was first practiced in Ancient Babylon around 2600 BC. In this era the priest, physician and pharmacist was the same person. The Arabs were the first to separate the art of pharmacy from physician and in the eight century they establish the first private pharmacy in Baghdad. When the European countries were exposed to Arabian influence, public pharmacies began to appear. However, it was not until about 1240 A.D. that pharmacy was separated from medicine.

3. Current global role of pharmacist

The role of the pharmacist is changing drastically with the traditional activities of the pharmacist such as extemporaneous compounding of medicines reducing and pharmacist becoming more like a walking encyclopedia for drugs, fulfilling the doctor's needs by giving advice and information on use of drugs, providing correct dosage forms, assuring the efficacy and quality of the dispensed or supplied medicinal products, formulating dosage forms and manufacturing drugs.

There has been a great transition in the profession and patient care has become the pillar of the practices. Now the pharmacy profession is not only related to dispensing and distribution of drugs or sometimes being regarded as a "glorified store keeper". A lot of societal and political influences and the development of new legislative instruments in most nations have paved the changes in the pharmacy profession that we are seeing today. Pharmacists now have a bigger role as global players and in the adoption of global standards so as not to be left out or left behind in the global race. This also has to be in line with global trends and forecasts for the pharmaceutical industry.

4. The basis of ethics for the pharmacy profession

Generally, the pharmacist is responsible for dispensing and compounding drugs or preparing suitable dosage forms for administration of drugs where overall these include patient pharmaceutical care in the clinical area, manufacturing, community pharmacy and research, with the latter including collection, identification, purification, isolation, synthesis, clinical trials, standardization and quality control of medicinal substances. All the above responsibilities of a pharmacist formed the basis for the requirement of a set of ethics guidance.

5. Pharmacy legislation

Pharmacy legislation generally includes the regulations for the practice of pharmacy, the sale of medicines and poisons, the dispensing of narcotics and other drugs of abuse, sale of drugs, quality assurance on drug manufacturing and advertising of drugs and medical devices. A pharmacist should dispense drugs within the provisions of the legislation of the country in which he practices. Such legislation recognizes the national pharmacopoeia along with international pharmacopoeia such as the United States Pharmacopoeia (USP), European Pharmacopoeia (EP) and British Pharmacopoeia (BP). These pharmacopoeias define products used in the practice, the purity of the drug, dosages and strength, and ensuring the standard for drugs in term of quality, safety and efficacy. The World Health Organization (WHO) traditionally plays a very important role to ensure that drugs in the global market are safe and affordable by poorer nation and, along with that, encouraging developed nations to harmonize their standards requirement to facilitate drug accessibility.

6. Pharmacist in different clusters with different ethical issues

The areas of pharmaceuticals can be clustered according to practices and their ethical issues.

6.1 Ethical issues in clinical pharmacy practice

Ethical issues arise as part of daily practice in the clinical setup in hospitals.

6.1.1 Patients pharmaceutical care

Pharmaceutical care is the current practice in pharmacy where pharmacists are responsible in view of drug therapy for the purpose of achieving best outcomes that promote a patient's quality of life. Clearly there are ethical issues in this new development. Among others, the ethical issues in pharmaceutical care practice are patient confidentiality and privacy, patient autonomy, duty to warn, competencies in deciding the best medication to be procured.

On the confidentiality and privacy issues, there is a general duty recognised by professional ethical codes which apply to all health and social care staff and this also includes pharmacists and their staff. Respecting confidences between pharmacists and patients enables patients to disclose the sensitive information that pharmacists need to provide pharmaceutical care (Wingfield et al., 2004). Without an assurance that confidentiality will be maintained, patients may be less willing to disclose information, resulting in obstacles to effective pharmaceutical care.

The autonomy of a pharmacist is always influenced by the unavoidable physician-patient relationship. This autonomy interfaces with the ethics of a physician. Pharmacists are always in a conflict position weighing the patient's rights for information and the physician's ethics for non-disclosure. A good example will be the non-disclosure of the side effects of a drug by a physician, e.g. in the case of prescribing a cancer drug a physician may not want a patient to be informed of the side effects as this may lead to patient incompliance.

The above topic on autonomy is also closely related to the duty of the pharmacist to warn on pharmaceutical issues and products. Warning a patient has to be balanced with the doctor's instructions and a conflicting situation need to be avoided. It would be unethical for a pharmacist to directly advice against a doctor's instruction to a patient without first informing the doctor involved.

The pharmacist, as a health professional in systems where value for money is an issue, requires competencies in deciding the best medication. The pharmacist is involved with making decisions on which drugs to include on a national formulary and to set guidelines on which drugs are used in a national hospital setting. Pharmacists have an active role in this decision-making process so currently most pharmacy teaching institutions have a module termed pharmacoeconomics in their curriculum, in which students will be trained to consider all issues in deciding which is the most economical drug based on the current literature. Consideration will be given to quality of life. The aspects covered include minimization of drug costs, cost effectiveness of drugs, cost utility, cost benefit, overall cost of illness, cost consequences. These aspects form the economic analytic technique that provides valuable information to pharmacists in making suggestions on which drugs will be more economical overall. The International Society for Pharmacoeconomics and Outcomes (ISPOR) gives the following definition: "Pharmacoeconomics is the scientific discipline that evaluates the clinical, economic and humanistic aspects of pharmaceutical products, services, and programs, as well as other health care interventions to provide health care decision makers, providers and patients with valuable information for optimal outcomes and the allocation of health care resources. Pharmacoeconomics incorporates health economics, clinical evaluations, risk analysis, technology assessment, and health-related quality of life, epidemiology, decision sciences and health services research in the examination of drugs, medical devices, diagnostics, biotechnology, surgery, disease-prevention services." (ISPOR 2011).

Members of the decision-making team should not have personal vested interests in companies which manufacture drugs, e.g., owning stocks, research support, speaker's bureau.

6.1.2 Interaction with other medical professionals

Pharmacist in clinical practice have to work with nurses, doctors and other medical professionals and they are very much needed to give advice on the latest medications, drug substitution, drug costing and everything to do with drugs or related devices. Often, pharmacists do not work directly with the patient, but rather with other health care professionals to complement the patient's therapy. However, there are opportunities for pharmacists to see patients when accompanying physicians and nurses on ward rounds. This will be one of the ethical issues where pharmacist is there to assist the other professionals but not to comment on short comings involving other professionals on the therapy. Sometimes it is difficult to balance the two and pharmacists have to be professional in handling such matters. A substantial percentage of a pharmacist's daily work will be interacting with other health professionals and this has to be done in an ethical manner.

6.2 Ethical issues in community pharmacy practice

Community pharmacy traditionally had a drug product focus wherein the primary business emphasis has been on drug distribution. In recent years, this emphasis has evolved, resulting in pharmacy becoming a more patient centered profession which emphasizes a shared responsibility between the patient and pharmacist for optimal drug therapy outcomes. This section explores the ethical issues involved in modern community pharmacy practice and discusses the related ethical dilemmas.

6.2.1 Dispensing of drugs

Ethical dispensing of drugs, medicinal devices and other products presents part of the requirement for rational drug therapy. Dispensing is not merely giving away drugs just like a vending machine based on prescription issued by doctors. Pharmacists need to dispense a drug professionally where this practice will include giving information of drugs in use or new drugs, information on side effects, drug interactions with other drugs or with food, recommendations on drug administration for unique situations (e.g. renal failure), information regarding appropriate drug dosage based on various factors (e.g. renal clearance, weight), information on national drug registration, information on administration of drugs, warnings, precautions and contraindications, storage conditions and stability of drugs.

Pharmacists can implement their right to refuse to dispense based on professional judgment. It is specified in the many national pharmacy laws that a pharmacist can refuse to dispense, if in the pharmacist's professional judgment, the prescription does not seem to be valid, or if filling the prescription as written could cause inadvertent harm to the patient. The basis of of a "pharmacist's professional judgment" will be based on the pharmacists' knowledge of the safety of the drug where ethically pharmacist should not allow hazard to the patient's health and welfare or anything which might result in suffering.

The question is whether a pharmacist has the right to refuse to dispense based on personal beliefs. An example could be whether a Muslim pharmacist can refuse to dispense products derived from pork. This issue can only be investigated by reading in-depth the relevant religious beliefs because, as a human being, a pharmacist also has freedom of speech. This may not be a good example as pork material can be used by Muslims in emergency cases if there is no substitute. Another question that arises will be whether it is ethical to dispense a substitute based on religious beliefs.

On the issues of online dispensing there are a lot of controversies and legal issues. According to Constance HF, Hawkin EW and Steven M in Mayo Clinic Prod. 2004 all these issue fall into 3 major categories: independent internet-only sites, online branches of pharmacies and sites representing partnerships among neighbourhood pharmacies. They further elaborate that potential benefits of online pharmacies include increased access, lower transaction and product costs and greater anonymity. However, they also stressed that online pharmacies have generated controversies, including the use of "cyberdoctors" on some sites, the dispensing of drugs without prescriptions from other sites and the import of prescription medications. Although some online pharmacies are legitimate and likely provide benefits to patients, other online pharmacies engage in questionable practices. Several nations have tried to regulate internet pharmacies as there are potential risks along with benefits of using online pharmacies. All these issues go back to the ethics of the pharmacist involved in such dispensing.

6.2.2 Prescribing of Pharmacy Only Medicines (POM)

Based on the classification of certain drugs by certain nations, pharmacist can dispense without a doctor's prescription or indirectly the public can buy preparations directly over the counter from pharmacist. This involves ethical practice by pharmacist where such sales should be in line with the authority guidelines to ensure public safety. Dispensing has always been the pharmacist's right but in some nations where the number of pharmacist is small the idea of the pharmacist's dispensing right is not implemented. In such countries the doctor does the prescribing and the dispensing together. Pharmacists in these countries are given the right to dispense without prescription certain categories of drugs to the public. In such conditions the ethics of the pharmacist is very much needed so that medicines that are being sold do not harm the public. For example in some countries certain drug like oral contraceptives (OCs) are being sold without prescription by pharmacists. In such cases the pharmacist has to input a high level of ethical control so that OCs are not simply sold to youngster and this matter needs judgment from the pharmacist to ensure safety to the public and to avoid certain drugs being abused. Another issue is the abusive use of local steroids in dermatological preparations, as these preparations are regulated as POM by some nations and they are readily available through pharmacies, and the pharmacist has to apply their knowledge to advise the public on the use of such preparations.

Pharmacists have a professional obligation as the gatekeepers of non-prescription medicines. The public may be able to obtain readily-accessible efficacious medicines through a pharmacist but the sale has to be immediately supervised and given proper information and consultation by the pharmacist. In most nations this direct dispensing by a pharmacist will carry legislative responsibilities to the pharmacist for ensuring proper sales and recording. Some countries use the term "immediate supervision" in their regulation on pharmacist dispensing without prescription. This means that pharmacist has to be available in the premise where the dispensing was done.

This category of drugs (non-prescription drugs) is one of criteria which drive toward self medication. With this classification of drugs, the public can buy preparations that were previously available only on prescription. A study in the UK shows that sales of over the counter medicines are now equivalent to a third of the NHS drugs bill (B. Colin and B. Alison 1996). This study also showed that over any two week period, nine out of 10 adults in the UK will experience at least one ailment, where non-prescription medicines are used to treat one in four of these episodes. There is a move toward smart self-medication and some governments throughout the world see self medication as a way of shifting some of the cost of healthcare onto consumers.

6.2.3 Patients' drug consultations

Pharmacists are professionals, expected to be very knowledgeable on drugs and to give drug consultations to the public in an ethical manner. Drug consultation is needed to advise patients on drug selection, drug dosage, understanding drug effects and side effects and interaction of drugs with other drugs or with food. This consultation can also include advice on general health information, management of certain conditions, diet and exercise. Some nations regulate the layout of a community pharmacy to allocate an area for patient counseling and drug information. It is globally accepted that drug consultations are free.

Public may request consultation with a pharmacist during their visit to a community pharmacy. Pharmacist cannot assume that they know the patient's best interest, the patient need to provide information and assist the pharmacist in their decision making (Latif, 2001).

Conventionally a pharmacist needs to keep records on all drug transaction as required by national laws. These records are among others for a pharmacist to monitor the dispensing of drugs to provide accountability when it comes to drug recall. These records will also capture the trends of drug usage and of prescribing by physicians. Community pharmacists also need to maintain individual records for patients who frequently consult them for advice on their medication. In such cases pharmacists have to ensure that personal medical records are kept private and confidential. All such records should be handled personally by the pharmacist and the national Code of Conduct of Pharmacist needs to address this matter to ensure pharmacists respect such confidentiality. Any breach of the confidentiality requirements is a great breach of ethical conduct. If in the case where records are kept electronically using a computer, the pharmacist has to ensure and validate the security of the records. This can be done by adoption of certain software which uses a password for access and amendments to records will be recorded in the history so that the old record can easily be retraced.

6.2.4 Extemporaneous pharmaceutical preparations

Extemporaneous preparations are products, which are dispensed immediately after preparation and not kept in stock (Pharmaceutical Inspection Convention, 2008). Extemporaneous preparations can be considered as unlicensed drugs where this preparation does not by law need to be concerned with quality, stability, bioavailability, efficacy and safety. As there are no published standards in the compendium, the standard depends very much on the professionalism of the pharmacist preparing the preparation. The pharmacist is referred to as the person who is skilled in the art. The uniformity of content, selection of safe excipients and stability issues form the challenges in the preparation of extemporaneous products. Dispensing of extemporaneous preparations of various dosage forms needs to have some ethical guidance, where this will involve the following issues:

6.2.4.1 Assuring quality in extemporaneous preparations

Extemporaneous preparations are preparation of dosage forms for particular patient consumption. There is no requirement of submission for registration with the authority so the quality of this type of preparation relies solely on the pharmacist and ethical issues on this matter need to be considered. Efforts to improve the quality of licensed and manufactured medicines are always on the agenda of pharmaceutical authorities but extemporaneously prepared products are still needed. So the pharmacist has the responsibility of ensuring that accurate and effective doses and dosage forms are made to achieve optimal drug therapy for certain groups like children and the elderly. Extemporaneous preparation is one facet of unlicensed drug use which can be a modification to commercially manufactured products such as the preparation of suspensions or powders from tablets or a preparation from individual raw materials where the pharmacist needs to be guided with some information from a reliable compendium. Extemporaneous preparation is popular in paediatric cases as this is to overcome the problems associated with the lack of approved medicines for children (Giam and McLachan, 2008).

Among the compendiums concerned with extemporaneous to which the pharmacist ethically has to refer are: the European Pharmacopoeia (2007), which is used as an official regulation for extemporaneous preparations, the British Pharmacopoeia (BP), the United States Pharmacopeia (USP), the Australian Pharmacopoeia Formulae (APF) and Martindale (Glass and Haywood, 2006). General instructions of the extemporaneous preparation are presented in Medicinal Products for Human and Veterinary Use: Good Manufacturing Practice (Eudralex, 2007) and in PIC/S Guide to good practices for the preparation of medicinal products in healthcare establishments (Pharmaceutical Inspection Convention, 2008).

6.2.4.2 Stability issues of extemporaneous preparations

Issues affecting the stability of extemporaneous preparations may include degradation of the drug, evaporation of the vehicle, loss of uniformity, change of appearance, change of bioavailability and toxicity caused by degradation products. There should be some form of stability evidence for extemporaneous preparations.

The stability of extemporaneous preparations refers to the chemical and physical characteristics of the preparation and the microbiological conditions (US Pharmacopeia, 2008). The shelf life of an extemporaneous preparation is predicted after an accelerated stability study has been carried out but more often extemporaneous preparations are given arbitrary shelf-lives (Costello et al., 2007). It is pertinent for a pharmacist to ensure that an extemporaneous formulation will remain within its physical, chemical and microbiological set conditions during storage for a specified time (Florence and Attwood, 2006). A short expiry period may be inconvenient for patients but a long expiry date will put the product and the user in jeopardy.

It is clear that it is the responsibility of the pharmacist to at least perform a stability study and predict the shelf life of a commonly prepared extemporaneous preparation so that there is evidence to support the quality of the extemporaneous preparation.

6.3 Ethical Issues in manufacturing of pharmaceutical products

Pharmaceutical manufacturers not only manufacture drugs and dosage forms but they also develop, produce, and markets drug licensed for use as medications. Manufacturers are subjected to a variety of laws and regulations regarding the manufacturing, testing and ensuring quality, safety and efficacy and marketing of drugs.

6.3.1 Quality assurance in pharmaceutical manufacturing

As defined by most documents, quality assurance is a system of actions devoted to ensure, with reasonable confidence, the quality of a product for its intended purpose. Ethics are pertinent to quality assurance as the person involved strives by taking actions to meet quality level goals, which contributes to quality assurance.

Generally we can make the assumption that the quality assurance concept covers all matters that individually or collectively influence the quality of a product. Generally, the keynotes of quality assurance are: quality systems are the foundation for effective management of an organization; quality systems are based on the philosophy of prevention; quality systems address the whole business process; quality systems consist of structured documentation to provide control; quality systems ensure a complete record of what you have done and complete documentation of what to do. With these keynotes, clearly quality assurance needs high ethical conduct from a pharmacist in order to truly build quality into pharmaceutical products.

Pharmaceuticals quality assurance can be divided into four major areas: quality control, production, distribution and inspections. To support quality assurance, there are standards and guidelines developed to supervise the procedures toward achieving quality. Quality assurance will have guidance documents for production, testing and distribution of pharmaceuticals. Among the documents are: guidelines for good manufacturing practices; guidelines for regulatory approval of pharmaceuticals; prequalification of pharmaceuticals, laboratories and supply agencies; and guidelines on quality control testing. Different countries will have their own set of guidelines which will be in line with their own national pharmaceutical legislations. For international purposes (usually for export of pharmaceutical products) international guidelines prepared by the World Health Organization (WHO) or the International Conference on Harmonisation (ICH) will be adopted.

6.3.2 Good manufacturing practice

Good Manufacturing Practice (GMP) is part of a quality system covering the manufacture and testing of pharmaceutical dosage forms or drugs. It outlines the aspects of production and testing that can impact the quality to a product. GMP ensures that quality is built into the product from the first step of production, not merely testing for quality at the end of the production line. GMP is concerned with both production and quality control (QC), where QC is a set of actions to test the acceptability of the raw materials, processed materials, final product and packaging material.

The basic requirements of GMP include: ensuring that all manufacturing process are clearly defined, systematically review for consistency in the production of a medicinal product of the required quality and specification and ensuring that critical steps of the manufacturing process and significant changes to the process are validated.

To ensure GMP achievement, the responsible person such as a pharmacist needs to ensure that the organization has adequate and appropriately qualified and trained personnel, adequate premises and space for the manufacturing, suitable equipment for the intended purpose with a proper plan for preventive maintenance, correct materials, containers and labels being used to maintain the quality of the product, approved procedures and instructions for manufacturing and suitable storage and transport.

A pharmacist in the GMP organization should also make sure that a system is available to recall any batch of the product, from sale or supply if a defect has been identified in a batch. Pharmacists also need to ensure that complaints about marketed products are examined, the causes of quality defects investigated and appropriate measures taken in respect of the defective products and to prevent reoccurrence of the defect. Pharmacists need to implement corrective and preventive measures to assure defects are corrected and do not happen again in future.

Clearly a pharmacist is key personnel in view of GMP. This key personnel status needs a profession and a person with high integrity. So, as a pharmacist is a professional, governed by a professional body, they should practice within the code of ethics in GMP facilities.

6.3.3 Good storage practice and good distribution practice

The quality of pharmaceutical products can be affected by a lack of adequate control over numerous activities which occur during the storage and distribution process. Good Storage Practice (GSP) is also part of a quality system covering the storage of pharmaceutical dosage forms or drugs. It outlines the aspects of storage that can impact the quality of a product after it has been manufactured in GMP manner. Good Distribution Practice (GDP) is also part of the quality system which covers the distribution of pharmaceuticals. The storage and distribution process should also be emphasized with regard to the need for establishment, development, maintenance and control over the activities involved. The guidelines for storage and distribution will assist in ensuring the quality and integrity of pharmaceutical products in all aspects of distribution and storage. In order to maintain quality, safety and efficacy, every activity in the storage and distribution of pharmaceutical products should be carried out according to the principles of GMP, GSP and GDP.

The storage and distribution of pharmaceutical products are different in different countries. There may also be differences between systems used in the public and the private sectors. All persons involved in any aspect of the storage and distribution of pharmaceutical products are ethically responsible, starting from the premises of manufacture to the point of supply to health establishments, such as private pharmacies, hospitals and clinics for supply to the patient. So all parties involved in trade and distribution, pharmaceutical manufacturers, including manufacturers of finished products, brokers, suppliers, distributors, wholesalers, traders, transport companies and forwarding agents, need to abide by the national requirements on storage and distribution.

One important issue in GSP and GDP is the cold chain system in handling and storage of certain categories of pharmaceuticals that require refrigeration, e.g. certain vaccines. A cold chain is a concept of supply chain which emphasized on temperature-controlled which is to ensure that the low temperature chain is unbroken according to series of storage and distribution activities by maintaining a given temperature range. For pharmaceuticals, it is used to ensure the shelf life of products such as vaccines or other products which is temperature sensitive. Cold chain is important in the supply of vaccines to clinics in hot climates. Disruption of a cold chain may develop consequences of non-effectiveness vaccination. Cold chain is part of the good manufacturing practice (GMP) which all pharmaceuticals and biological products are required to follow. Cold chain must be validated to ensure that there is no negative impact to the safety, efficacy or quality of the pharmaceuticals. GMP requires that all processes that might impact the safety, efficacy or quality of the drug substance must be validated, including storage and distribution of the drug substance. A cold chain should be managed ethically by validation of a distribution process, which among the needs of cold chain are logistics of shippers (providing tracking of the status of the temperature maintenance with prove of documentation), using refrigerator trucks, refrigerated warehouses, products are insulated with specialized packaging, temperature data loggers and tags to help monitor the temperature history of the products while shipping or kept in warehouse or while they are kept by the pharmacist or physician, every step of the cold chain needs to be properly recorded. From this brief explanation on cold chain we can see clearly that those who manage pharmaceutical which requires cold chain need to be very ethical to ensure the efficacy and safety of the product. There can be serious breach of ethics if a product is being reinstalled with a new tag when its original tag has shown that the cold chain had been broken.

6.3.4 Ethics of pharmacists in handling product complaints and product recalls

Most nations regulate that all complaints and other information concerning defective pharmaceutical products, must be carefully investigated according to written procedures. The pharmacist in charge of complaints is responsible for initiating the investigation immediately. The investigation shall be documented in writing. If a product defect is discovered or suspected in a batch, the pharmacist should also take into consideration to determine whether other batches are also affected. If the defect is life threatening, the pharmacist should take immediate action by all reasonable means, whether in or out of business hours to recall the product.

Pharmacists should always be prepared for product safety alerts, where products can be in a situation of not conforming to the safety specifications. When there is a risk of significant hazard to consumers from a product which has been distributed in the market, pharmacists should take the responsibility of disseminating the safety alert through mass communication media available, including newspapers, radio and television. Fast action should be taken according to documented procedures to remove the defective product from sale or use. Clearly the pharmacist is responsible to establish a system to recall products known or suspected to be defective from the market promptly and effectively. The pharmacist should be ethical, when deciding the fate of the recalled products. The recalled product may be reworked if it meets appropriate standards and specifications. The recalled product should be destroyed if the condition of the product casts doubt on its safety, identity and quality. The pharmacist has to be ethical in making all these decision where priority should be given to the safety of human beings and not to monetary considerations.

6.4 Ethical issues on wholesale, supply, import and export of drugs

Wholesale, supply, import and export are all actions on distribution of drug which are controlled by permits and licenses. Pharmacists trusted with such permits or licenses need to show a high level of ethics as drugs can be diverted to illicit channels for misuse and drugs can also be counterfeited and patient safety is always at stake. The ethical need in this issue is paramount for categories of drugs which have tendencies to be abused. Dangerous drugs such as morphine, fentanyl or pethidine or psychotropic substances such as diazepam or barbiturates and their derivatives need to be dealt with a high level of ethics as pharmacists are trusted as guardians to these highly abusive drugs and the tendency of being abused by pharmacists is high as the sales can be very lucrative to the pharmacist.

Globally most nations are member of the International Narcotic Control Board (INCB), United Nations (Vienna). As stipulated by the INCB, import and export of dangerous drugs or psychotropic substances need to be authorized by the importing nation and also the exporting nation following the procedures set by the INCB. An import authorization will be issued to the pharmacist by the competent authority of the importing country. Upon receiving a copy of the import authorization from the competent authority of the importing country, the competent authority of the exporting country will issue an export authorization to allow the exporter to export the product. It will be unethical for a pharmacist not to follow the requirement of the INCB in terms of import and export of such drugs.

6.5 Ethical issues in research and clinical trials

Good Research Practice (GRP) should ensure that research is well-planned, appropriately designed and ethically approved. The requirement of ethics committee approval is a stringent requirement for medical related research where there may be use of animal or human subjects. Approval is needed from the institutional review board (IRB) or institutional ethics committee (IEC) of the respective establishment on research involving humans or human tissues, medical records or surveys of certain research issues. In the US, an IRB is a board, a committee, or a group of people formally designated by an institution like hospitals, academic medical centers, government units, and others engaged in conducted or supported health research activities involving human subjects, to review research involving humans as subjects. An IRB has the authority to approve, modify, or disapprove related research activities. Upon approval, IRBs must conduct periodic reviews of such research. In the US, all IRB must have not less than five members with varying backgrounds and each member must be sufficiently qualified through the experience and area of expertise. The membership should also be as diverse as possible in term of race, gender, and cultural backgrounds. IRB should not include member who has conflict interest, except on special cases where needed. All IRBs must include at least one member who are in scientific areas and at least one member who are in nonscientific areas. Some nation do not have IRB but instate they have institutional ethics committee (IEC) with similar set up of members and function as an IRB.

Drug development research is one of the main activities of a pharmaceutical company involved in research. Modern drug development follows the following key stages: program selection (choosing the disease target), identification and validation of the drug target, assay development, identification of a lead compound, optimization of the lead compound, identification of a drug candidate, preclinical study (a broad study encompassing animal studies, toxicity studies and pre-formulation studies), clinical trials on human subjects, registration and release of the drug to the market and follow-up monitoring (adverse drug reaction reporting). Generally, pharmaceutical companies will invest more on research for drugs which are likely to be more lucrative in their sales. Usually those diseases suffered by people in developed nations will be more attractive for the pharmaceutical companies. For example, not much research is being carried out by pharmaceutical companies on drugs for AIDS as the vast majority of AIDS sufferers are from the third world such as those from the African continent. Ethically this is not right but the pharmaceutical companies need to pay back the money which has been spent on research.

6.5.1 Preclinical research

Preclinical research involves studies of a drug before it is approved for studies on humans. These studies are designed to collect data at the earliest stage (such as cell culture study) to confirm activity. Among the studies can be spectroscopic studies to identify the chemical structure of the drug-like compound and animal studies using wide-ranging doses of the study compound to obtain preliminary effectiveness and toxicity data along with determination of the pharmacokinetics of the new compound in animal models and to predict the pharmacokinetics in humans. Preclinical studies will assist pharmaceutical companies to decide whether a drug candidate has scientific merit for further development.

Preclinical studies must adhere to Good Laboratory Practice (GLP). The International Conference on Harmonisation (ICH) guidelines for GLP should be adopted by nations as a standard. An ethical issue here is for the pharmacist involved in the study to abide by the guidelines stipulated. Furthermore the use of animals in the studies needs to have clearance from the animal ethics committee. Animals are used to study the toxicity, including studies on organs that are targeted by the new compound, as well as studies on any long-term carcinogenic effects or any adverse effects on the reproduction system. Some nations have even made it compulsory to study the effects on genes. Information collected from preclinical studies is important so as to ensure the follow-up clinical trials on humans is safe and there are no unexpected adverse effects. Although animal studies in pharmaceutical research have been reduced in recent years both for ethical and cost reasons, most research will still involve animal-based testing for the need of similarity in anatomy and physiology that is required for diverse product development.

Another important component in preclinical studies where pharmacists play a very important role are the pre-formulation studies. Pre-formulation is a branch of pharmaceutical sciences that utilizes biopharmaceutical principles in the determination of physicochemical properties of a drug substance. Commonly evaluated parameters of the new compound in pre-formulation studies are solubility, ionization constant (pKa), partition coefficient (Log P), dissolution behaviour, stability, solid state properties such as crystal forms/polymorphs, water sorption behavior, surface properties, particle size and shape, and other mechanical properties. In depth pre-formulation studies are needed as this will determine the end dosage form of the new drug. Data from these studies will be used to decide whether the dosage form will be an oral solid dosage form or an intravenous dosage form or any other best route of administration. At this stage the dosage form determination is pertinent as the new compound will be given to humans for the purpose of clinical trials.

6.5.2 Clinical trials for new drugs

In the study of a new chemical entity for the purpose of developing a medicine, clinical trials in humans are among the last steps to be carried out. They will only be started after the chemical entity has gone through extensive preclinical studies and found to be fit and proper for human use and a dosage form for humans has been developed. Clinical trials enable us to evaluate and assess the effectiveness of a new medicine in the treatment of a particular condition and also help to disclose possible side effects. Before such a new medicine can be approved by the regulatory authorities, it must be proven to be efficacious and safe in the targeted patient population.

Clinical trials will involve human subjects as volunteers so it is of paramount importance to ensure the safety and well-being of these volunteers and that all trials are conducted in accordance with global ethical principles. Clinical trials deal with human beings so the human rights and dignity of people participating in clinical trials need to be protected. Clinical trials follow a set of global accepted protocol in line with the requirements of the national health authority. All clinical trials need to be approved by the national institutional ethics committee (IEC) in the country where they are carried out. These global standards are not to be compromised. Clinical trials must be conducted in the same way all the time, no matter where in the world and by whom they are carried out.

Investigators must carefully select the subjects to participate to have the right profiles, obtain informed consent from each subject and take steps to ensure the well-being of the subjects throughout and after the trial. Clinical trials must undergo independent scientific and ethical review and approval and are subject to audit by the national authorities during or after the trial. All clinical trial results must be made publicly available.

Clinical trials on humans are usually carried in a randomised and blinded manner, so that subjects, and in some trials also the investigators, do not know if the treatment that the subjects are receiving is the new drug or the control treatment. These trials may use placebo as a control. This means that test subjects are randomised to receive either the new medicine or a placebo. This technique is termed as "randomized double-blind, placebo-controlled trial" where a group of the subjects are given the treatment, another group are given placebo, and neither the researchers nor the subjects know which is which until the study ends. For over the years researchers have established that for most types of trials, only a randomized double-blind, placebo-controlled study can answer the question whether a drug in a trial really work. Commonly ethics committees have reservations on the use of a placebo as it is seems to be very unethical to give subjects with the disease condition a placebo. So placebo will only be used if ethically acceptable for example if the new treatment is given in addition to the existing treatment, a placebo can be used to mask whether the participant is receiving the new treatment and the existing treatment, or just the existing treatment.

Generally clinical trials are clustered into four different phases (Spilker, Bert., 1984). Phase I involves the first testing of a new compound in human subjects for the purpose of establishing the tolerance of healthy human subjects at different doses, defining its pharmacologic effects at anticipated therapeutic levels and studying its absorption, distribution, metabolism, and excretion patterns in humans. Phase I can involved 100-200 subjects. Generally Phase 1 studies will assess the most common acute adverse effects and examine the doses that patients can take safely without serious side effects. At this stage we begin to clarify what happens to the new drug when it is in the human body. Question like how is it metabolized, how much of it (or a metabolite) gets into the blood and various organs, how long it stays in the body, and how the body gets rid of the drug and its effects, will hopefully be answered.

In Phase II, controlled clinical trials with the new medicine give information on its potential usefulness and short term risks. A relatively small number of patients, usually no more than several hundred subjects, are enrolled in phase II studies. At this stage the efficacy of the medicine is fully established and the dose response relationship is established. This phase usually includes an active comparator (as control).

Phase III involves general studies of the new medicine safety and effectiveness in both hospital and outpatient settings. This phase gathers information on the medicine's effectiveness for the specific indications, determines whether the medicine causes a broader range of adverse effects than those exhibited in the phase I and II studies and identifies the best way of administering and using the drug for the purpose intended. If the drug is approved for registration, this information forms the basis for deciding the content of the product label. Phase III studies can involve several hundred to several thousand subjects.

Phase IV generally takes place after the medicine has been approved for marketing. It comprises market surveillance studies as required by authorities globally. As this phase takes place after market authorisation is given, it determines the effectiveness and safety of the product in an even wider variety of populations. It may also be conducted on request from authorities as a condition for market authorisation approval to address specific safety issues. The extensiveness of the clinical trial has to be implemented together will the global requirement of other human right declarations.

Clinical trials should always be conducted according to global human rights declarations such as the Declaration of Helsinki, the Nuremberg code, the Belmont report and the International Conference on Harmonisation (ICH) guidelines for Good Clinical Practice. The interest and well-being of the trial subjects should always prevail over the interest of science, society and commerce. Clinical trials will only be conducted if they can be scientifically and medically justified and potential benefits outweigh potential risks. Children should only be included in a trial if there is no other research alternative.

Subjects participating in a clinical trial should, after the study has finished, be offered the best possible treatment, at the discretion of the investigator. Everyone has to ensure transparency of clinical trials and clinical trial results for the good of humanity.

It is interesting to know the historical development of ethics consideration in using human subjects for clinical trials. In the early twentieth century there were no regulations regarding the ethical use of human subjects in research and no requirements for ethics approval or an institutional review board (IRB) whatsoever. An eye opener to the need of ethics consideration for use of human subjects is the well known Nuremburg tragedy where during the world war, German physicians conducted medical experiments on thousands of concentration camp prisoners without their consent and most of the subjects of these experiments died. A military tribunal for war crimes and crimes against humanity was set up and as a result of the trial the Nuremberg Code was established in 1948. The Nuremburg Code states that subjects should give consent and that the benefits of research must outweigh the risks.

Realizing the need of ethical implementation on the use of human subjects the World Medical Association established the Declaration of Helsinki in 1964, guiding medical doctors involved in research using human subjects. The declaration stated that all research with humans should be based on the results from laboratory and animal experimentation, research protocols should be reviewed by an independent committee prior to initiation, informed consent from research participants is compulsory, research should be conducted by qualified individuals and the risks of research should not exceed the benefits.

It is ironical that the Declaration of Helsinki did not stop the unethical use of human subjects in the case of Tuskegee Syphilis Study conducted by the U.S. Public Health Service between from 1932 to 1972. Six hundred low-income African-American males, 400 of whom were infected with syphilis, were monitored for 40 years. Free medical examinations were given; however, subjects were not told about their disease. Even though a proven cure (penicillin) became available in the 1950s, the study continued until 1972 with participants being denied treatment. Many subjects died of syphilis during the study. The study was stopped in 1973 by the U.S. Department of Health, Education, and Welfare only after its existence was publicized and it became a political embarrassment.

In response to this, the United States created a Commission for the Protection of Human Subjects, which drafted the Belmont Report in 1979, a foundational document for the ethics of research with human subjects in the U. S. The Belmont Report stated the basic ethical principles that should assist in resolving the ethical problems that surround the conduct of such research: respect for persons, beneficence and justice. These three basic principles were used to enforce the need for informed consent, the need to assess the risks and benefits and the need for proper selection of subjects.

Clearly the Helsinki Declaration, Nuremberg Code and the Belmont Code are pertinent to the pharmacy profession as pharmaceutical companies are parties who initiate clinical trials for their new drugs or new formulations. Pharmaceutical companies will engage Clinical Trial Organization (CRO) to manage the clinical trial. The CRO will ensure that the doctors involved abide by all the requirements of Good Clinical Practice which encompasses the criteria stipulated in the declarations and codes.

7. Ethical marketing of pharmaceutical products

Pharmaceutical organizations are made up of pharmacists who are governed by their professional bodies, so each pharmacist has a duty to uphold an ethical relationship within the business. They are required by their code of conduct to care for the health and safety of human beings. A question frequently raised is how pharmacists can ensure that ethical standards are upheld when pharmaceutical companies have large investments and stakeholders to protect. Because of this several nations not only regulate pharmacists as people that should abide by the code of ethics but also pharmaceutical companies.

It is very misleading to believe that ethical equates to lawful and it may be untrue to think that by being lawful an organization, activity or person is ethical. Look around us, many unethical practices are entirely lawful. For example mercurial soap used for skin whitening is unlawful to be marketed in all developed nations but some of these nations allow the manufacture of such products for export markets. Some nations allow manufacturing of patented product but still the act of producing patented products is unethical.

Pharmaceutical companies use the service of sales representatives in marketing their products. These sales representatives need to be adequately trained and possess sufficient medical and technical knowledge to present information about the products in an accurate and responsible manner. The sales representative should not only be able to provide accurate information, but should also not to exaggerate the capabilities of the product. He or she should be able to talk about the property of the product or the mode of action of the drug and possible side effects. It is a well known practice for a sales representative to give free samples to physicians. All these free sample need to be accounted for by way of recording by the pharmaceutical company so that the traceability of the product can be maintained for the purpose of product recall. The practice of giving other gifts by pharmaceutical companies to physicians is unethical. A good example is giving free overseas trips under the pretence of sponsorship for attending conferences or workshops. In this case the pharmaceutical companies and the physician can both be guilty of misconduct under their own code of conduct.

Pharmaceutical organizations must not only see how much profit can be made but also how ethical is the profit that is made. Pharmaceutical organizations in many countries have developed a code of pharmaceutical marketing practices to be adopted by their members. Among the recommendations is that all marketing activities under the code must conform to existing and relevant government legislation governing the practice of the pharmaceutical industry. The code stresses that members should have good management of complaints which documented procedures of investigation and with set time frames for processing each complaint lodged. Corrective and preventive outcomes of complaint investigation should also be documented. Generally the code also outlines all possible issues in disseminating accurate, fair and objective information to the medical and allied professions so that rational prescribing decisions can be made. Members are required to follow high standards of conduct and professionalism in the marketing of pharmaceutical products. Such a code should also have ethics committee to hear, receive and deliberate on all breach of ethics issue. This committee should set penalties for breach of the code and publish the names of companies, which have been found to be in breach of the code, which may result in them suffering adverse publicity.

8. Pharmacists role in complementary & alternative medicines

Complementary and alternative medicines are health practices that have the component of pharmaceutical preparations, dietary supplements, and traditional forms of health practice such as acupuncture, Chinese medicine, homeopathy, etc. Very recently complementary and alternative medicines have become a important component of health care regimens. Many countries legitimized complementary and alternative medicines by registering them so that their quality and safety can be controlled as their use by the public are unavoidable. However there is no way that the authority can ascertain their efficacy. Lacking the efficacy component their registration requirement is of a lesser standard than conventional medicines. Although lack of scientific and poor efficacy of complementary and alternative medicines, there is some evidence (or the only evidence for efficacy of complementary and alternative medicines) found such as the use of cranberry for urinary tract infections and St. John's Wart for depression. Most of the other claims on the effectiveness of complementary and alternative medicines are not evidence based.

Pharmacists are in an ethical dilemma in the use of complementary and alternative medicines. As health care professional pharmacist are expected to provide a high level of unbiased, evidence based health care (Applebe et al., 2002), while their business side is expected make profit. Pharmacist's professionalism and business roles are in conflict with the sale of alternative medicines. Great consideration need to be given as Pharmacists selling complementary and alternative medicines in their pharmacies will give credibility to these products and to some extent will promote their usage. Pharmacist has the responsibility to provide the factual advice for patients who seek out these products. Pharmacists can play the role in counseling for the use of complementary and alternative medicines is to ensure the health and safety of patients is not jeopardized. All counseling should adhered to the principles of evidence based medicine and honestly informing the customers of the unproven therapies but respect have to also be given to the customer's the beliefs and their autonomy to make decisions regarding their own treatment while at the same time pharmacist offer professional advice. There are cases where the complementary and alternative medicines are completely contradictory to the principles of modern medical science and a good example is the Homeopathy treatment concept. This contradiction with all of basic medical sciences must be taken into consideration. Globally the ethical issues pharmacists face on complementary and alternative medicines are being handled appropriately according to the Code of Conduct or Code of Ethics of particular nation and based on the global perception, pharmacists is one of the most trusted health professionals.

9. Ethics in advertising

Previously, in most nations the advertising and promotion of ethical pharmaceutical products was mainly carried out for physicians and pharmacists. However from the early 1990s, companies began direct-to-consumer (DTC) advertising. DTC advertisements were used in some developed nations to inform the public that physicians had a new treatment to help them treat certain diseases. The advertisements did not mention the name of the products, but rather, they asked patients with specific problems or symptoms to see their physician for advice. This sort of DTC advertisement was quite popular in the United States. The question will be is it ethical to influence the public to ask their physician on drug prescribing.

In the middle 1990s DTC advertising in the United States went through another stage where such advertisements were allowed for magazines and newspapers where the name of the product and its indication for use are also mentioned, but such DTC advertising on television or radio only mentions either the name of the product or the indication for the product as advertisement space is limited in such media. The happening in the US led to the liberalization of drug advertisement to the general public and led the way for other nations to follow. Some small nations or developing nations are skeptical about allowing such advertisement for prescription drugs due to concerns over public perception. These nations feel that their citizens are not yet ready for such liberalization of drug advertisement.

The United State Authority has ruled that this technique of advertising can be very effective because it increases awareness among the public that a new treatment or drug is available and influences them to talk to their doctors. The Americans have now moved forward to allow DTC advertising of prescription products on the television and radio, in which advertisers can now mention both the name of the product and indications with a condition that the main precautions or warnings are also given. This has led to a revolution in the way prescription products are advertised on television.

In addition to this, advertising and promotion to physicians, seminars and symposia goes on as usual. Sales representatives are as active as ever calling on doctors, pharmacists and other health-care professionals. These representatives will give information about their companies' products, how to use them, the possible side effects and the different dosage forms available. They also give away samples to physicians and these samples are sometimes used to initiate treatment for a new patient or, in some cases, to provide medication for a patient who cannot afford to buy it. Ethical questions are always being asked about whether it is ethical to give away free samples or to give medicines for free give to the customers. Some nation have regulated against giving away free samples for certain categories of prescription drugs.

A number of pharmaceutical control authorities feel that pharmaceutical companies are spending too much on advertising and promotion and some even regulate the amount of revenue to be used for advertising as a form of control. The expenditure on advertisements is actually paid by the consumers as broadly advertised drugs will be more costly to the consumers.

10. Ethics in intellectual property

Broadly, intellectual property means the legality which results from intellectual activity in the industrial, scientific, literary and artistic fields (WIPO Handbook). Intellectual property law in all nations generally aims at safeguarding creators and other producers of intellectual goods and services by granting them certain time-limited rights to control the production and sales. Pharmacists and the pharmaceutical companies and organizations are very familiar with this intellectual property concept as it forms the basis of pharmaceutical invention control. If a pharmaceutical company develops a new drug, the company will enjoy the exclusive right to produce and market the product until the patent expires. This concept is known to be well respected among the pharmaceutical manufacturers. It is very unethical for a pharmaceutical product to be copied before the expiry of the patent.

There are also irresponsible companies in nations where patent law is not well respected, who will produce a copy of the product and sell the product through the black market. The pharmacist in the retail pharmacy has to be ethical not to deal with any product which has infringed the patent requirements. The authority in a nation also needs to enforce the patent law in order to be more protective of patents.

From the point of view of the patent owner, they also have to be ethical in getting profits from the patented product. We are witnessing today a global issue whereby patent owners do not totally let go of patents upon their expiry. Certain multi-national companies (MNCs) try to prolong the exclusive right to the product by re-patenting the same product with some modification. Sometimes it looks like it is well planned by the company from the beginning when the first patent was filed. The company, knowingly, first patented an inferior product formulation and then patented a superior product formulation on the expiry of the first patent and the same company enjoyed the exclusivity again. The public will then be deprived of a generic product. A good example will be a situation where a pharmaceutical company first patents a capsule dosage form (where this dosage form is quite bulky) and then patents a tablet dosage form (a smaller, more favourable dosage form) upon patent expiration with a novelty claim in terms of extra processing which is different from the normal text book technique of making tablets. This is unethical conduct since such a case can only be solved through court cases to nullify the patent and this can be very expensive. It is a serious breach of ethics and the patent authority should be more vigilant in preventing such unethical behaviour. They should seriously scrutinize the novelty or the inventive nature of the second formulation.

11. Conclusion

Ethics in the area of pharmaceuticals which concern the pharmacist as a person and the pharmaceutical company as a corporate body is experiencing evolution, where pharmacy practice is different today than it was previously. Pharmaceutical innovation and technology advancement has shaped the pharmaceutical industry and pharmacists themselves and the need of solid strong ethics to be embedded into the pharmacist as an individual which will then form the organization of pharmaceutical with high ethical values. Ethics and pharmacy at large must be sensitive and responsive to an unavoidably changing environment.

12. References

Applebe G. E., Wingfield J.,Taylor L. (2002). Practical Exercises in Pharmacy Law and Ethics. Pharmaceutical Press, London.

Constance H. F, Hawkin E. W, Steven M. (2004). Controversies and Legal Issues of Prescribing and Dispensing Medications Using the Internet. Mayo Clin. Proc. ,79, 188-194.

Costello I., Long P.F., Wong I.K., Tuleu C., Yeung V. (2007). Paediatric drug handling. Pharmaceutical Press, Cornwall.

Eudralex: Volume 4 -Medicinal Products for human and veterinary use: Good Manufacturing practice.

European Pharmacopoeia. (2007). supplement 6.1 to the 6th edition. Council of Europe, Strasbourg, France.

Giam J.A., McLachlan A.J. (2008). Extemporaneous product use in paediatric patients: a systematic review. Int. J. Pharm Pract. 16, 3-10.

Glass B.D., Haywood A. (2006). Stability considerations in liquid dosage forms extemporaneously prepared from commercially available products. J. Pharm. Pharmaceut. Sci. 9, 398–426.

International Society for Pharmacoeconomics and Outcomes Research (ISPOR), 2011. Brief Definition of Pharmacoeconomics , at, http://www.ispor.org/Terminology/Default.asp

Latif D. (2001). The Relationship Between Pharmacists'Tenure in the Community Setting and Moral Reasoning. Journal of Business Ethics, 31(2), 131–141.

Martindale (2002). The complete drug reference, 33rd ed. Ed. Sweetman SC, Pharmaceutical Press, London.

MSH and WHO (Management Sciences for Health and World Health Organization). 1997. *Managing Drug Supply.* 2nd ed. West Hartford, CT: Kumarian Press.

Nuremberg Code, The. *Reprinted in Trials of War Criminals before the Nuernberg Military Tribunals under Control Council Law* No. 10, Vol. 2, pp. 181-182. Washington, D.C.: U.S. Government Printing Office, 1949. Also reprinted in Ethics and Regulation of Clinical Research, 2d ed., by Robert J. Levine, pp. 425-426. Baltimore: Urban and Schwarzenberg, 1986.

Pharmaceutical Inspection Convention (2008). PIC/S Guide to good practices for the preparation of medicinal products in healthcare establishments.

Spilker, Bert., Guide to Clinical Trials. Raven Press, New York, 1991 *The Belmont Report (1978) Ethical Principles and Guidelines for the Protection of Human Subjects of Research.* Washington, D.C.: U.S. Government Printing Office, DHEW Publication No. (OS) 78-0012. Reprinted in Federal Register 44 (April 18, 1979): 23192.

Wingfield J., Bissell P., Anderson C.(2004). The Scope of Pharmacy Ethics—An Evaluation of the International Research Literature, 1990–2002', Social Science and Medicine 58, 2383–2396.

World Medical Association (1989). "Declaration of Helsinki." As amended by the 41st World Medical Assembly, Hong Kong, September 1989.

World Intellectual Property Organization. The concept of Intellectual properties. WIPO Intellectual Property Handbook: Policy, Law and Use

7

Placebo Use in Depression Research: Some Ethical Considerations

Ybe Meesters, Martine J. Ruiter and Willem A. Nolen
University Medical Center Groningen, Dept. Psychiatry, Groningen, The Netherlands

1. Introduction

Placebo use in depression research is under discussion. The World Medical Association (WMA, 1964; 2008) states in their Declaration of Helsinki that ethical principles for medical research involving human subjects are important. Accordingly, benefits, risks, burdens and effectiveness of new interventions must be tested against those of the best current proven intervention, with some exceptions.

Some present-day ethical reviewing committees do not allow the use of placebos in depression research. On the other hand, some government organizations (among them the Food and Drug Administration in the USA and the European Medicines Agency in Europe) will not authorize new interventions or medications in healthcare systems unless their effectiveness has been proved in randomized placebo-controlled trials.

In this chapter, we will discuss the principle that the use of a placebo condition is not allowed in depression research if an effective treatment is already available. This issue is important in research investigating the effects of new interventions or medications. In this chapter, considerations for and against placebo use, based on the literature, will be discussed. It will be argued that the use of a placebo condition is ethically defensible.

2. History

Public knowledge of the abuse of humans for scientific research led to legislation to end this abuse. The best-known example of abuse is that by the Nazi physicians during the Second World War, who forced prisoners to participate in their investigations. In 1946 a trial started at Nuremberg against 23 physicians and their assistants (the so-called "Doctors' Trial") for their actions as criminals of war. In 1947, this trial led to the Nuremberg Code, in which, for the first time, conditions and criteria were formulated describing what makes research on humans acceptable (López-Muñoz et al., 2007; Markman and Markman, 2007). The Nuremburg Code pays special attention to informed consent and freedom of choice for participants', the relation between the study's risks and benefits and the participant's right to end their collaboration at any time (Rice, 2008). In 1964 the World Medical Association presented the so-called Declaration of Helsinki, which since has been updated several times, which the most recent update in Seoul in 2008 (http://www.wma.net/en/30publications/10policies/b3/). Apart from this most countries have their own regulations.

At first it was widely believed that the abuse of humans for research purposes only occurred in countries with oppressive totalitarian regimes and not in modern democratic societies. In reality, however, unethical investigations in which research harmed the participants have also been performed in Western countries. An example is a study from the USA, in which the researchers withheld an effective treatment for a long time (1932-1972) from humans suffering from syphilis (Brandt, 1978). The discovery of these facts resulted in the Belmont Report (National Institutes of Health, 1979) which provides guidelines for research with humans in the USA.

Recently, more unethical behaviour of physicians from the same period (±1940) was published. In Guatemala, US Public Health Service researchers deliberately infected patients with syphilis, without their consent, which led to the death of at least 83 of them. A presidential US commission investigated this abuse. According to an announcement of the chair of the Presidential Commission for the Study of Bioethical Issues (2011), an extensive report with recommendations will appear at the end of 2011 to assure the public that today's scientific and medical research is conducted in an ethical manner.

3. Legislation

The Declaration of Helsinki is used worldwide as a starting point to establish the acceptability of research on humans. In addition to this declaration most countries have their own legislation. In the Netherlands, the Law on Medical Scientific Investigation in Humans (Wet Medisch-Wetenschappelijk Onderzoek; WMO, 1998) decides, among other things, that every investigation with humans must be approved by an ethical reviewing board (Institutional Reviewing Board (IRB)).

According to the Declaration of Helsinki, it is important that the physician acts in the patients' best interest and that participating in a research study will not adversely affect the health of the patients serving as research subjects.

In the placebo discussion section 32 of the Declaration of Helsinki is highly important:

'The benefits, risks, burdens and effectiveness of a new intervention must be tested against those of the best current proven intervention, except in the following circumstances:

- *The use of placebo, or no treatment, is acceptable in studies where no current proven intervention exists; or*
- *Where for compelling and scientifically sound methodological reasons the use of placebo is necessary to determine the efficacy or safety of an intervention and the patients who received placebo or no treatment will not be subject to any risk of serious or irreversible harm. Extreme care must be taken to avoid abuse of this option.'*

4. Depression

Lots of people feel down or sad sometimes. These feelings are usually short-lived and only last a few days. Patients suffering from a depression are in a state of low mood for a long time (at least 14 days) with a loss of interest and pleasure in daily activities. Depression is a common, but serious illness which influences daily life and well-being negatively and which can be accompanied by a number of symptoms. Depressed people may feel sad, anxious, empty, hopeless, pessimistic, helpless, worthless, guilty, irritable, or restless. They may lose interest in activities that once were pleasurable, experience loss of appetite or overeating, or problems concentrating, remembering details or making decisions. They may also contemplate or attempt suicide. Insomnia, excessive sleeping, fatigue, loss of energy or aches, pains and digestive problems resistant to treatment may be present (National Institute of Mental Health, 2011).

Depression interferes with daily life and well-being. Most people who experience depression need treatment to get well again. Medications, psychotherapies, and other methods are effective treatments for patients with depression.

A classification system, used by psychiatrists and psychologists worldwide, is the Diagnostic and Statistical Manual of Mental Disorders, Fourth Edition (DSM-IV, American Psychiatric Association, 1994). The DSM-IV formulates criteria and distinguishes different forms of mood disorders by severity and duration. Patients with a:

- major depressive disorder or major depression suffer for at least two weeks from a combination of symptoms interfering with their ability to work, sleep, study, eat, and enjoy once-pleasurable activities. Major depression is disabling and prevents a person from functioning normally. Some people may experience only a single depressive episode in their lifetime, but more often they will have multiple episodes.
- dysthymic disorder, suffer from long-term symptoms. These symptoms are not severe enough to disable the patient but can prevent normal functioning or feeling well. People with dysthymia may also experience one or more episodes of major depression during their lifetimes.
- minor depression have symptoms that do not meet the full criteria for major depression for two weeks or longer.

Different forms of mood disorders are specified on the basis of the symptoms, for example:

- Patients with a psychotic depression are severely depressed and also suffer from a form of psychosis, such as experiencing delusions or hallucinations
- A seasonal affective disorder (SAD) is characterized by the onset of depression during the winter months, when there is less natural sunlight. This type of depression generally disappears in spring and summer. An effective treatment for SAD is light therapy.
- A bipolar disorder (also known as manic-depressive disorder) is characterized by cyclic mood changes – from extreme highs (mania) to extreme lows (depression). There are two types of this disorder. A Bipolar I Disorder is mainly defined by manic or mixed episodes lasting for at least seven days, or manic symptoms that are so severe that the affected person needs immediate hospital care. The depressive episodes usually last for two or more weeks. The symptoms of mania or depression must be a major change from the person's normal behavior. A less severe disorder is a Bipolar II Disorder which is defined by a pattern of depressive episodes shifting back and forth with hypomanic episodes, but with no full-blown manic or mixed episodes (American Psychiatric Association, 1994; National Institute of Mental Health, 2008).

5. Effectiveness of evidence-based treatments for depression

Antidepressants are considered effective in patients suffering from depression and are recommended in guidelines, such as those of the APA guidelines in the US (American

Psychiatric Association, 2006), the NICE guidelines in the UK (National Institute for Health and Clinical Excellence, 2004) and the Multidisciplinary Guidelines for the Treatment of Depression in the Netherlands (Landelijke Stuurgroep Multidisciplinaire Richtlijnontwikkeling in de GGZ, 2010), as evidence-based treatments. Nevertheless, their effectiveness is sometimes questioned (Enserink, 1999; Kirsch et al., 2008; Turner et al., 2008). Some authors state that the effects of antidepressants are not much higher than those of sophisticated placebos (Antonuccio et al., 1999; Kirsch & Sapirstein, 1998).

Moreover, the placebo effects of treatments are not just found in controlled studies, but are also present in clinical practice, even when no placebo is given (Finniss, et al. 2010).

Treatment modalities other than medication are also relevant to this placebo discussion. For example, light treatment is highly effective as a treatment for seasonal affective disorder (SAD) (Pail et al., 2011) and according to the multidisciplinary guidelines mentioned above it is the treatment of first choice. A meta analysis by an APA work group shows that the effects of light treatment in SAD are comparable to the effects of treatment of non-seasonal depressions with antidepressants (Golden et al., 2005). In a recent study, Lieverse et al. (2011) found that bright light treatment was more effective than a placebo (dim light) in the treatment of non-seasonal depressions in the elderly. The authors stated that in this population, light treatment had the same effect as anti-depressants in the treatment of non-seasonal depressions.

Notwithstanding these studies, the Swedish government is still unconvinced of the effectiveness of light treatment, and is still waiting for a large placebo-controlled study to be conducted. Without such a study it does not want to recognize and approve the therapeutic value of light treatment (SBU, 2007).

An important problem is that the working mechanism of light treatment is still unknown (Meesters & Van den Hoofdakker, 1998). There is no clear methodologically justified placebo condition available for light treatment. For this reason, in light treatment research different placebo-like conditions have been used, such as imaginary light (Richter et al., 1994), invisible light (Meesters et al., 1997), extra-ocular light (Koorengevel et al., 2001), low-intensity light (Lieverse et al., 2011) or sometimes a placebo totally unrelated to light, such as a deactivated ion generator (Desan et al., 2007). Reponses to these 'placebo' conditions varied from 36% to 46.6%.

It is also unknown what other factors, such as attention and accompaniment or healthcare system-related aspects like referral and reimbursement play a role in the therapeutic effects of light treatment (Reesal & Lam, 1999).

6. Pros and cons of placebo use in depression research

As is the case in other more or less controversial issues, there are supporters and opponents of placebo use in the field of depression research. Opponents of placebo-controlled studies object to the fact that a physician in the placebo condition does not offer the best-known effective treatment to the patient or withholds this treatment for a certain amount of time (Miller, 2000; 2002; Pużyński, 2004; Waring, 2008).

According to the Declaration of Helsinki participants of placebo-controlled studies should not run any more risks than they would in accepted regular treatments. These risks are increased mortality, permanent serious harm and reversible but serious harm or greater discomfort than usual. The greatest risk for humans with a severe depression is without doubt the risk of suicide. Khan et al. (2000) used data from the Food and Drug Administration (FDA) concerning 45 placebo-controlled studies on 7 new medicines against depression. 34 out of 19,639 participants committed suicide and 130 made a suicide attempt. There was no difference in the rates of completed suicides or suicide attempts between patients who were given active medication versus those who received the placebo. The same conclusion was drawn in a meta analysis of data from the European Medicines Agency (EMA) (Storosum et al. 2001). This indicates that the fear of an increased suicide risk for participants receiving a placebo condition is not evidence-based. A possible reason for this is that most studies exclude patients with an increased suicide risk (those with previous attempts and suicidal ideation).

Nevertheless, there may be other risks than suicide, for example the consequences of a long-lasting depression, such as the risk of losing a job, or a serious deterioration of the relationship with a partner or children. These possible consequences have not been well investigated (Kim, 2003; Kim and Holloway, 2003).

In efficacy studies of new medicines or other interventions such as light treatment in an acute phase of depression these risks would seem limited. The duration of these studies is short: mostly 6-8 weeks. If the effects are disappointing, a different, hopefully more effective treatment can be tried. Therefore, participation in a placebo-controlled study can result in a delay of up to 1 or 2 months before patients receive an active treatment.

Perhaps placebo-controlled studies in more vulnerable groups need more careful attention, as in the case with patients with very severe depression (e.g. psychotic depression), patients with increased suicide risks, or patients with depressions during pregnancy. So far, in the last group, very little evidence of an effective treatment has been found. Depressions are known to be harmful for the mother and her unborn child, so it is important to find a treatment that is harmless to both. This treatment has to be both safe and effective. Nowadays many physicians advice against antidepressant medication because of the uncertain effects on the unborn child. In those cases the mood disorder continues to exist, and this is also harmful. Therefore, it is stated that well-conducted placebo-controlled studies are ethically justified in these cases (Coverdale et al., 2008).

An alternative for a placebo-controlled study is a study in which the new intervention is compared with an active comparator. The power of this type of study is far less than that of a placebo-controlled study. Therefore more participants have to be recruited for the study to be able to draw conclusions. When the new intervention turns out to be ineffective, more patients will have received an ineffective treatment as compared to those in a placebo-controlled study (Berk, 2007).

Supporters of placebo-controlled studies first of all argue that it is the only way to show the efficacy of a new intervention. Even if a study shows that a new intervention does not differ in its effects from a well-known existing treatment, there is no evidence for the efficacy of the new intervention if no placebo condition is included. In the field of psychiatric research there are many similar studies. We mention two examples here.

In a study with people suffering from a bipolar I disorder it was found that in maintenance treatment the effectiveness of divalproex was not different from lithium. Without a placebo-arm the conclusion might have been that divalproex is as effective as lithium, the effectiveness of which had been shown in previous studies. However, in this study, both active drugs were not more effective than placebo (Bowden et al. 2000).

In another study with patients suffering from a major depressive disorder it was shown that the use of hypericum (St John's Wort) did not differ from the well-known antidepressant sertraline. However, in this study too, the effects of the two treatments were not different from placebo (Hypericum Depression Trial Study Group, 2002).

In both of these studies it was impossible to show the efficacy of the new interventions (divalproex, hypericum) because they were not more effective than placebo, despite the fact that they did not differ from the two well-known existing interventions with proven activity (Quitkin, 1999; Kupfer & Frank, 2002). This conclusion would not have been possible if there had not been a placebo condition. The reasons for such 'failed trials' are open to speculation. Differences in study populations may be a cause of this:

- Participants may have been suffering from another type of bipolar disorder or depression.
- Patients may have been less severely ill.
- Patients may have been included who had been treated unsuccessfully before with the same or similar drugs.
- There may have been high drop-out rates.
- Other methodological limitations may have been present.

In studies investigating the effects of new interventions in the treatment of depression it is therefore necessary to include a placebo condition in the research program.

Secondly, it should be clear that the response to placebo in depression research varies widely, between 10% to 50% and in the majority of studies amounts to at least 30%. Moreover, the response to placebo has increased over time with about 7% per decade (Walsh et al., 2002; Kahn et al., 2005). In a recent meta analysis of 96 studies it was found that 68% of the effects of antidepressants could be explained as a placebo effect (Rief et al., 2009). If we keep these data in mind, it is clear that in new studies it is impossible to rely on a 'historic placebo condition', i.e. the response to placebo in previous studies.

Third, restriction or prohibition of placebo-controlled studies makes it impossible to discover more effective treatments or treatments with fewer disturbing side-effects. In a placebo-controlled study the conclusion that the side-effects of a new intervention can be distinguished from the side-effects of an existing treatment must be inconclusive. However, without a placebo condition the question about the effectiveness of the new intervention must be inconclusive (Baldwin et al. 2003).

Fourth, another reason to defend the use of placebo is that new medicines or interventions can have unknown safety issues. It is argued that for the treatment of major depression with a new medicine, placebo-controlled studies are the best way to take these aspects into account. Abandoning placebo controlled studies would lead to less certainty about the safety and effectiveness of the new medicines (Dunlopp and Banja, 2009).

Finally, in placebo-controlled studies fewer participants are needed to show an effect when compared with studies without a placebo condition. Therefore, studies with a placebo are less expensive and easier to realize. This is the point of view of forums in the field of depression research. These forums, such as the European Expert Forum on Ethical Evaluation of Placebo-Controlled Studies in Depression (Baldwin et al., 2003; Adam et al., 2005), the National Institute of Mental Health (NIMH, Hyman and Shore, 2000), the National Depressive and Manic-Depressive Association (Charney et al., 2002) and the FDA

(Laughren, 2001) made a plea for the inclusion of a placebo condition in depression research and emphasized its necessity. The Council of Ministers of the European Union and the EMA (Helmchen, 2005) will not exclude the possibility of placebo-controlled studies.

7. The role and functioning of medical ethical reviewing boards

A medical ethical reviewing committee or institutional review board (IRB) is an independent committee which has been appointed to approve, monitor, and review biomedical and behavioral research involving humans. Its purpose is to protect the rights and welfare of the research subjects. The aim of an IRB is to review critical functions (scientific, ethical, and regulatory) for research on humans.

Few researchers would question the usefulness or necessity of medical ethical reviewing committees. In the Netherlands it is unlawful (WMO, 1998) to start an investigation with a new intervention in humans without the approval of an ethical reviewing committee. Sponsors, funding agencies, insurance companies and scientific journals (see among others Touitou, et al., 2006) demand this approval before giving their support to studies involving humans or publishing results.

This makes an IRB a very powerful institution. Its opinion about a study is decisive for whether this study will be conducted. The way in which the IRBs are fulfilling their mission is not always satisfactory for the investigators in the research field (Van Santvoort, et al., 2008). Sometimes bureaucratic procedures or excessive attention to futilities cause serious delays (Alberti, 2000; Nicholl, 2000; Tully et al., 2000; Giles, 2005; Keith & Koocher. (2005); Martinson et al., 2005; Dingwall, 2006; Yawn et al., 2009). Another problem may arise when different IRBs judge research projects in different ways. Sometimes IRBs in the same country judge differently (Van Teijlingen et al., 2008).

However, there are more basic reasons leading to dissatisfaction, such as the rejection of placebo conditions on principle by IRBs. There are several international guidelines in relation to placebo-controlled research, varying from a total ban to acceptance with some restrictions (Ehni en Wiesing, 2008). The IRBs' requirements for non-invasive intervention research differ widely in different European countries (Hearnshaw, 2004) despite the fact that all European countries have signed the Declaration of Helsinki.

Another complicating issue is the opinion of major government institutions. Although many countries endorse the Declaration of Helsinki, these institutions have formulated regulations which are not in line with this declaration. For example, the FDA in the United States has decided that clinical trials performed outside of the USA no longer have to conform to the Declaration of Helsinki when they are used to support applications for products in the USA and follow other standards (DHHS, Food and Drug Administration 2008). This decision has been heavily criticized (among others: Lurie and Greco, 2005; Normile, 2008; Goodyear et al., 2009). Also, the European legislation as implemented by the EMA has been criticized as favouring the interests of pharmaceutical companies above patients' interests (Garattini et al., 2009). These discrepancies in rules and opinions can be rather confusing, especially in multicenter studies in different countries with different IRBs.

The discrepancy between everyday practice together with the requirements of FDA or EMA and the Declaration of Helsinki is also criticized as being unethical (Rothman & Michels, 1994; Michels & Rothman, 2003).

In the Netherlands the acceptance of a placebo condition is also under discussion in those cases where an existing treatment is available in the field of psychiatric research. Most IRBs act pragmatically, however. If an existing treatment is available, a placebo condition is often accepted if the burdens and risks for the patient are limited and a clear rule for the collaboration on the study is included in the protocol in the case of deterioration of the patient's condition, together with the proposal to the patient, that, if necessary, they will receive the best-practice treatment after finishing their collaboration to the study (Nolen and Engberts, 2000).

8. Discussion

For a long time the opinion among experts has been that well-known treatments for depression are effective. This opinion is becoming less pronounced. For instance, a meta-analysis showed that antidepressants were only effective in placebo-controlled studies with patients who had severe depressions. No differences with placebos were found in patients with mild depressions. Moreover, antidepressants (and other treatments used for depression) are not effective in all patients (Kirsch et al, 2008; Whitaker, 2010). Up to 40-50% of patients do not show a satisfactory response. Therefore, the development of new, effective treatments is highly important, which makes the use of placebo-controlled study designs still necessary.

In this chapter it was argued that there is no sufficient evidence for a treatment of depression where the treatment outcome is the sole result of this treatment. According to the exceptions mentioned in section 32 of the Declaration of Helsinki, there is currently no best proven intervention available. This justifies the use of a placebo condition in depression research if the effectiveness of a new intervention or medicine is the subject of research. Besides, methodological reasons make it unacceptable to initiate research into new interventions for the treatment of depressions without a placebo condition. This is caused by the great heterogeneity of depression and the unpredictability of a placebo response. Therefore, it can be argued that the inclusion of a placebo condition in efficacy studies with new compounds or interventions to treat depression should be a standard rather than an exception (Meesters, et al., 2009, 2010). As long as new compounds or interventions are not more efficacious than standard treatments, the only way to show their efficacy is to compare them with a placebo. Performing efficacy studies without a placebo and taking the risk that no valid conclusions can be drawn at the end of the research because a placebo arm is missing, can also be considered unethical.

9. Acknowledgements

The authors are grateful to Josie Borger for the improvement of the English.

10. References

Adam D., Kasper S., Muller H.-J & Singer; 3rd European Expert Forum on Ethical Evaluation of Placebo-Controlled Studies in Depression. (2005): Placebo-controlled trials in major depression are necessary and ethically justifiable. European Archives of Psychiatry and Clinical Neurosciences 255: 258-260

Alberti K.G.M.M. (2000): Multicentre research ethics committees: has the cure been worse than the disease? British Medical Journal 320: 1157-1158

Antonuccio D.O., Danton W.G., DeNelsky G.Y., Greenberg R.P. & Gordon J.S. (1999): Raising questions about antidepressants. Psychotherapy & Psychosomatics 68: 3-14
American Psychiatric Association (1994): Diagnostic and Statistical Manual of Mental Disorders, Fourth Edition, Washington DC: American Psychiatric Association
American Psychiatric Association (2006): American Psychiatric Association Practice Guidelines for the Treatment of Psychiatric Disorders Compendium 2006. Arlington: American Psychiatric Association
Baldwin D., Broich K., Fritze J., Kasper S., Westenberg H. & Möller H.J. (2003): Placebo-controlled studies in depression: necessary, ethical and feasible. European Archives of Psychiatry and Clinical Neurosciences 253: 22-28
Berk M. (2007): The place of placebo? The ethics of placebo-controlled trials in bipolar disorder. Acta Neuropsychiatrica 19: 74-75
Bowden C.L., Calabrese J.R., McElroy S.L., Gyulai L., Wassef A., Petty F., Pope H.G., Chou J.C.-Y., Keck P.E., Rhodes L.J., Swann A.C., Hirschfeld R.M.A.& Wozniak P.J. (2000): A randomized, placebo-controlled 12- month trial of divalproex and lithium in treatment of outpatients with bipolar I disorder. Archives of the General Psychiatry 57: 481-489
Brandt A.M. (1978): Racism and research: the care of the Tuskegee Syphilis Study. Hastings Cent Rep 8: 21-29
Charney D.S., Nemeroff C.B., Lewis L., Laden S.K., Gorman J.M., Laska E.M., Borenstein M., Bowden C.L., Caplan A., Emslie G.J., Evans D.L., Geller B., Grabowski L.E., Herson J., Kalin N.H., Keck P.E. Jr, Kirsch I., Krishnan K.R., Kupfer D.J., Makuch R.W., Miller F.G., Pardes H., Post R., Reynolds M.M., Roberts L., Rosenbaum J.F., Rosenstein D.L., Rubinow D.R., Rush A.J., Ryan N.D., Sachs G.S., Schatzberg A.F., Solomon S.; Consensus Development Panel (2002): National depressive and manic-depressive association consensus statement on the use of placebo in clinical trials of mood disorders. Archives of General Psychiatry 59: 262-270
Coverdale J.H., McCullough L.B. & Chevenak F.A. (2008): The ethics of randomized placebo-controlled trials of antidepressants with pregnant women. A systematic review. Obstetrics & Gynecology 112: 1361-1368
Desan P.H., Weinstein A.J., Michalak E.E., Tam E.M., Meesters Y., Ruiter M.J., Horn E., Telner J., Iskandar H., Boivin D.B.& Lam R.W. (2007): A controlled trial of the Litebook light-emitting diode (LED) light therapy device for treatment of Seasonal Affective Disorder (SAD). BMC Psychiatry 7:38
DHHS Food and Drug Administration (2008): 21 CFR part 312. Human subject protection; foreign clinical studies not conducted under an investigational new drug application. http://www.regulations.gov?fdmspublic/component/main?main=DocumentDetail&o=0900006480537f08
Dingwall R. (2006): Confronting the anti-democrats: the unethical nature of ethical regulation in social science. Medical Sociology online 1: 51-58
Dunlop B.W.& Banja J. (2009): A renewed, ethical defence of placebo-controlled trials of new treatments for major depression and anxiety disorders. J Med Ethics 35: 384-389
Ehni H.-J.& Wiesing U. (2007): International ethical regulations on placebo-use in clinical trials: a comparative analysis. Bioethics 22: 64-74
Enserink M. (1999): Can placebo be the cure? Science 284: 238-240
Finniss D.G., Kaptchuk T.J., Miller F.& Benedetti F. (2010): Biological, clinical, and ethical advances of placebo effects. The Lancet 375: 686-695
Garattini S.& Bertele V. (2009): Ethics in clinical research. Journal of Hepatology 51: 792-797

Giles J. (2005): Researchers break the rules in frustration at review board. Nature 438: 136-135

Golden R.N., Gaynes B.N., Ekstrom R.D., Hamer R.M., Jacobsen F.M., Suppes T., Wisner K.L.& Nemeroff C.B. (2005): The efficacy of light therapy in the treatment of mood disorders: a review and meta-analysis of the evidence. American Journal of Psychiatry 162: 656-662

Goodyear M.D.E., Lemmens T., Sprumont D. & Tangwa G. (2009): The FDA and the Declaration of Helsinki. A new rule seems to be more about imperialism than harmonisation. British Medical Journal 338: 1157-1158

Hearnshaw H. (2004): Comparison of requirements of research ethics committees in 11 European countries for a non-invasive interventional study. British Medical Journal: 328: 140-141

Helmchen H. (2005): Ethische Implikationen plazebokontrollierter Prüfungen von Psychopharmaka. Der Nervenarzt 76: 1319-1329

Hyman S.E. & Shore D. (2000): An NIMH perspective on the use of placebos. Biological Psychiatry 47: 689-691

Hypericum Depression Trial Study Group (2002): Effect of hypericum perforatum (St John's Wort) in major depressive disorder. JAMA 287: 1807-1814

Keith-Spiegel P., Koocher G.P. (2005): The IRB paradox: Could the protectors also encourage deceit? Ethics & Behavior 15: 339-349

Khan A., Warner H.A.& Brown W.A. (2000): Symptom reduction and suicide risk in patients treated with placebo in antidepressant clinical trials. Archives of General Psychiatry 57: 311-317

Khan A., Kolts R., Rapaport M.H., K.R.R. Krishnan, Brodhead A.E.& Brown W.A. (2005): Magnitude of placebo response and drug-related differences across psychiatric disorders. Psychological Medicine 35: 743-749

Kim S.Y.H. (2003): Benefits and burdens of placebos in psychiatric research. Psychopharmacology 171: 13-18

Kim S.Y.H.& Holloway R.G. (2003): Burdens and benefits in antidepressant clinical trials: a decision and cost-effectiveness analysis. American Journal of Psychiatry 160: 1272-1276

Kirsch I.& Sapirstein G. (1998): Listening to Prozac but hearing placebo: a-meta analysis of antidepressant medication. Prevention & Treatment 1: 0002a

Kirsch I., Deacon B.J., Huedo-Medina T.B., Scoboria A., Moore T.J.& Johnson B.T. (2008): Initial Severity and Antidepressant benefits: a meta-analysis of data submitted to the Food and Drug Administration. PLoS Medicine 5(2): e45

Koorengevel K.M., Gordijn M.C.M., Beersma D.G.M., Meesters Y., Den Boer J.A., Van den Hoofdakker R.H.& Daan S. (2001): Extra ocular light therapy in winter depression: a double-blind placebo-controlled study. Biological Psychiatry 50: 691-698

Kupfer D.J.& Frank E., (2002): Placebo in clinical trials for depression. JAMA 287: 1853-1854

Landelijke Stuurgroep Multidisciplinaire Richtlijnontwikkeling in de GGZ (2010): Multidisciplinaire richtlijn Depressie (eerste revisie). Richtlijn voor de diagnostiek, behandeling en begeleiding van volwassen patiënten met een depressieve stoornis. Utrecht: Trimbos Instituut

Laughren T.P. (2001): The scientific and ethical basis for placebo-controlled trials in depression and schizophrenia: an FDA perspective. Eur Psychiatry 16: 418-423

Lieverse R., Van Someren E., Nielen M.M., Uitdehaag B.M., Smit J.H.& Hoogendijk W.J. (2011): Bright light treatment in elderly patients with nonseasonal major depressive disorder: a randomized placebo controlled trial. Arch Gen Psychiatry 68: 61-70

López-Muñoz F., Alamo C., Dudley M., Rubio G., García-García P., Molina J.D.& Okasha A. (2007): Psychiatry and political-institutional abuse from the historic perspective: The ethical lessons of the Nuremberg Trial on their 60th anniversary. Progress in Neuro-Psychopharmacology & Biological Psychiatry 31: 791-806

Lurie P.& Greco D (2005): US exceptionalism comes to research ethics. The Lancet 365: 1117-1119

Markman J.R.& Markman M., (2007): Running an ethical trial 60 years after the Nuremberg Code. The Lancet Oncology 8: 1139-1146

Martinson B.C., Anderson M.S.& De Vries R. (2005): Scientists behaving badly. Nature 435: 737-738

Meesters Y., Van Os T.W.D.P., Grondsma K., Veneman F., Beersma D.G.M.& Bouhuys A.L. (1997): Light box vs Light Visor; Bright white vs infrared or placebo light. SLTBR abstracts 9: 27

MeestersY.& Van den Hoofdakker R.H. (1998): Winterdepressie en lichttherapie II: prevalentie, etiologie, pathogenese en werkingsmechanisme. Tijdschrift voor Psychiatrie 40: 266-276

Meesters Y., Ruiter M.J.& Nolen W.A. (2009): Pleidooi voor placebogebruik in depressieonderzoek. Nederlands Tijschrift voor de Geneeskunde 153: A459

Meesters Y., Ruiter M.J.& Nolen W.A. (2010): Is het gebruik van placebo in onderzoek bij depressie aanvaardbaar? Tijdschrift voor Psychiatrie 52: 575-582

Michels K.B.& Rothman K.J. (2003): Update on unethical use of placebos in randomized trials. Bioethics 17: 188-204

Miller F.G. (2000): Placebo-controlled trials in psychiatric research: an ethical perspective. Biological Psychiatry 47: 707-716

Miller F.G. (2002): What makes placebo-controlled trials unethical? The American Journal of Bioethics. 2:3-9

National institute for Health and Clinical Excellence (2004): Depression: management of depression in primary and secondary care - NICE guidance London, Manchester: National institute for Health and Clinical Excellence

National Institute of Health (1979): The Belmont Report: Ethical Principles and Guidelines for the Protection of Human Subjects of Research, Report of the National Commission for the Protection of Human Subjects of Biomedical and Behavioral Research. http://www.hhs.gov/ohrp/archive/documents/19790418.pdf

National Institute of Mental Health (2008): Bipolar Disorder. http://www.nimh.nih.gov/health/publications/bipolar-disorder/complete-index.shtml

National Institute of Mental Health (2011):Depression. http://www.nimh.nih.gov/health/publications/depression/complete-index.shtml

Nicholl J. (2000): The ethics of research ethics committees. British Medical Journal 320: 1217

Nolen W.A.& Engberts D.F. (2000): Klinisch-wetenschappelijk onderzoek in de psychiatrie: ethische en juridische aspecten. Tijdschrift voor Psychiatrie 42: 575-584

Normile D. (2008): Clinical trials guidelines at odds with U.S. policy. Science: 322: 516

Pail G., Huf W., Pjerk E., Winkler D., Willeit M., Praschak-Rieder N.& Kasper S. (2011): Bright-light therapy in the treatment of mood disorders. Neuropsychobiology 64: 152-162

Presidential Commission for the Study of Bioethical Issues (2011): President's Bioethics Commission Concludes Investigation into 1940s STD Experiments in Guatemala. http//www.bioethics.gov/cms/node/280 (August 29, 2011)

Pużyński S. (2004): Placebo in the investigation of psychotropic drugs, especially antidepressants. Science and Engineering Ethics 10: 135-142

Quitkin F.M. (1999): Placebos, drug effects, and study design: a clinician's guide. American journal of Psychiatry 156: 829-836

Reesal R.T.& Lam R.W. (2001): Clinical guidelines for the treatment of depressive disorders II: Principles of management. Canadian Journal of Psychiatry 46 suppl. 1: 21S-28S

Rice T.W. (2008): The historical, ethical, and legal background of human-subjects research. Respiratory Care 53: 1325-1329

Richter P., Bouhuys A.L., Van den Hoofdakker R.H., Beersma D.G.M., Jansen J.H.C., Lambers P.A., Meesters Y., Jenner J.A., Van Houwelingen C.A.J.& Bos P. (1992): Imaginary versus real light for winter depression. Biological Psychiatry 31: 534-536

Rief W., Nestoriuc Y., Weiss S., Welzel E., Barsky A.J.& Hofmann S.G. (2009): Meta-analysis of the placebo response in antidepressant trials. (2009): Journal of Affective Disorder doi: 10.1016/j.jad.2009.01.029

Rothman K.J.& Michels K.B. (1994): The continuing unethical use of placebo controls. New England Journal of Medicine 331: 394-398

SBU (2007): Light therapy for depression, and other treatment of seasonal affective disorder. A systematic review. Revision of chapter 9 in SBU report treatment of depression (2004), no 166/2. Summary and conclusions in English. Report nr. 186

Storosum J.G. Van Zwieten B.J., Van den Brink W. Gersons B.P.& Broekmans A.W. (2001): Suicide risk in placebo-controlled studies of major depression. American Journal of Psychiatry 158: 1271-1275

Touitou Y., Smolensky M.H.& Portaluppi F. (2006); Ethics, standards, and procedures of animal and human chronobiology research. Chronobiology International 23: 1083-1096

Tully J.,Ninis N., Booy R, Viner R (2000): The new system of review by multicentre research ethics committees: prospective study. British Medical Journal 320: 1179-1182

Turner EH, Matthews AM, Linardatos E, Tell RA, Rosenthal R. (2008): Selective publication of antidepressant trials and its influence on apparent efficacy. N Engl J Med. 358:252-60

Van Santvoort H.C., Besselink M.G.H.& Gooszen H.G. (2008): Het verkrijgen van medisch-ethische goedkeuring voor een multicentrische, gerandomiseerde trial: prospectieve evaluatie van een moeizaam proces. Nederlands Tijdschrift voor de Geneeskunde 152: 2077-2083

Van Teijlingen E.R., Douglas F.& Torrance (2008): Clinical governance and research ethics as barriers to UK low-risk population-based health research. BMC Public Health 8: 396

Walsh B., Seidman S.N., Sysko R.& Gould M. (2002): Placebo response in studies of major depression. JAMA 287: 1840-1847

Waring D.R. (2008): The antidepressant debate and the balanced placebo trial design: an ethical analysis. International Journal of Law and Psychiatry 31: 453-462

Whitaker R. (2010): Anatomy of an epidemic. New York: Crown Publishers

WMA (1964; latest update: 2008): Declaration of Helsinki - Ethical Principles for Medical Research Involving Human Subjects. http://www.wma.net/en/30publications/10policies/b3/

WMO. Wet medisch-wetenschappelijk onderzoek met mensen (1998): Den Haag: Staatsblad 161

Yawn B.P., Graham D.G., Bertram S.L., Kurland M.J., Dietrich A.J., Wollan P.C., Brandt E.C., Huff J.M.& Pace W.D. (2009): Practice-based research network studies and institutional review boards: two new issues. J Am Board Fam Med 22: 453-460

Medical Ethics in Undergraduate Medical Education in Pakistan: Towards a Curricular Change

Ayesha Shaikh and Naheed Humayun
Federal Post Graduate Medical Institute,
Shaikh Khalifa Bin Zayed Al Nahyan Medical and Dental College,
Shaikh Zayed Medical Complex, Lahore,
Pakistan

1. Introduction

Curriculum is the skeleton of a subject, without which the muscles and organs will leave their place demolishing the structure. A well thought, well planned and a well written curriculum is the key to success for any subject. Curriculum of a subject, reflect the state of intellectual development of that population. Globalization has led to free availability of new ideas and information, which pours in continuously. It is, therefore, essential to update curricula by utilizing the recent developments and research evidence in the different fields of knowledge. Curriculum is defined as, "An educational plan that spells out which goals and objectives should be achieved, which topics should be covered and which methods are to be used for learning, teaching and evaluation"(Wojtczak, 2002). A more comprehensive definition states, "A curriculum is first of all a policy statement about a piece of education, and secondly an indication as to the ways in which that policy is to be realized through a program of action." It is added that, "it is the sum of all the activities, experiences and learning opportunities for which an institution or a teacher takes responsibility. He includes the formal and the informal, the overt and the covert, the recognized and the overlooked, the intentional and the unintentional education" (Coles, 2003).

"The curriculum is a complex network of physical, social and intellectual conditions that shape and reinforce the behavior of individual, and takes into consideration the individual's perceptions and interpretations of the environment in order to reinforce the learning objectives and to facilitate the evaluation procedures" (EduQnA.com, 2007). The first textbook on the subject of curriculum was published in early 20th century (Bobbitt, 1918).

In the 32nd UNESCO General Conference (UNESCO, 2003), the need to initiate and support teaching programs in ethics, bioethics and in all scientific and professional education was stressed by Member States, because of this, UNESCO initiated the ethics education program in 2004. Bioethics education for medical practice is essential because of continuous change; in medical policies and legislation on patient rights, complexity of health care systems and decision-making about emerging issues in clinical practice (McCrary, 2001). Research based arguments for the development and introduction of integrative medical humanities courses into the core curriculum were used. Ethics in contemporary medicine, is growing since the 1970's as shown by the increasing use of Institutional Review Boards for protection of human subjects, the establishment of hospital ethics committees, the demand of clinician ethicists and the integration of ethics into many medical education curricula (Evans & Macnaughton, 2001).

Pakistan is one of the underdeveloped capitalist countries, where the health care is curative and for the elite class. Literacy levels are low, medicine is taught in English, and nearly all prescribed textbooks are in English and for the West. The systems of health care and medical education are not in line with the real needs of the community and of the country (Zaidi, 1987). This is still the problem with our medical education that we focus on what others do rather than developing our own curriculum in the light of local needs.

The government of Pakistan approved the constitution of the National Bioethics Committee (NBC) in 2004. The purpose is to "promote and facilitate ethical health services delivery and health research" (Harvard School of Public Health, n.d.). The main role of the National Bioethics Committee (NBC) is of an advisory body dealing with all aspects of bioethics in the health sector of Pakistan. It also promotes and facilitates ethical health services delivery and health research. It has a supervisory and advisory role by linking with the ethical review bodies in organizations and institutions like the Pakistan Medical and Dental Council (PMDC), the Medical Training and Teaching Institutions and the recently constituted Good Clinical Practices (GCP) committee of the Ministry of Health's Drug Division. The committee has two sub-committees, the research ethics committee and medical ethics committee. NBC's medical ethics committee is responsible for the Bioethics teaching and training in medical education (Pakistan Medical and Dental Council, n.d.). Code of ethics for the doctors is given by PMDC (Pakistan Medical and Dental Council, n.d.).

Pakistan is a developing country aiming to provide excellence in Medical Education but still striving for achieving minimum standards of medical education. Undergraduate Medical education has given more attention during the first decade of twenty first century, which led to increased number of medical colleges all over Pakistan. The Pakistan Medical and Dental Council is the regulatory authority responsible for the recognition of medical colleges, setting and revising the medical education standards, developing and revising curriculum and registering the faculty.

The Pakistan Medical & Dental Council is a statutory body (Pakistan Medical and Dental Council, n.d.) constituted by the Federal Government under the Pakistan Medical & Dental Council Ordinance (Pakistan Medical and Dental Council, 1962). The Council is controlling it. One of the main objectives of the Council is to lay down the minimum standard of basic and higher qualifications in Medicine & Dentistry. "The Council has been empowered to prescribe; a uniform minimum standard of courses of training for obtaining graduate and post-graduate qualification, a minimum requirements for the content and duration of courses, admission criteria to the courses of training, the standards of examinations and method of conducting the examination for medical and dental studies" (Pakistan Medical and Dental Council, n.d.)

Curriculum Development, Review and Revision at Graduate and Postgraduate level is one of the major on-going activities of Higher Education Commission as provided under Section

(10) Sub-Section (V) of its Ordinance No.LIII, Government of Pakistan (Higher Education Commission, 2002). The Standard Operating Procedures for curriculum revision are followed by HEC in which the National Curriculum Revision Committee is responsible for the revision of the curriculum (HEC). HEC has developed procedures and guidelines for quality assurance and its enhancement for the university administration, quality enhancement cells and faculties for easier implementation (Batool & Qureshi n.d).

Human communities and professional organizations need to uphold values that are respected by the group as a whole, but there is a great concern about questions of "right" and "wrong" conduct. Same is the case with medical professionals. UNESCO mentioned the need to revise and update existing educational curricula as multifaceted, as a result large number of changes is occurring in the world. It provides a guide for managing curriculum changes with an objective to enhance educational quality and relevance. Six of the values that commonly apply to medical ethics discussions are;

- Autonomy means the patient has the right to refuse or choose their treatment.
- Beneficence means a practitioner should act in the best interest of the patient.
- Non-maleficence means "first, do no harm".
- Justice concerns the distribution of scarce health resources and it also deals with treating people with fairness and equality.
- Dignity means the patient (and the person treating the patient) has the right to be treated with respect and honor.
- Truthfulness and honesty - the concept of informed consent has increased in importance.

These values do not give answers as to how to handle a particular situation, but provide a useful framework for understanding conflicts. When conflict arises, the result is an ethical dilemma or crisis (UNESCO, n.d.). There are various ethical guidelines formulating the foundation of regulations regarding medical ethics; the Declaration of Helsinki (Kimmelman, Weijer & Meslin, 2009), ten points of Nuremberg code (U.S. National Institutes of Health, n.d.).

There are still deficiencies and gaps in the knowledge regarding ethics and code of conduct in different spheres of life. In Judeo-Christian and specially the Islamic teachings, one can get the acceptable conduct drive; explaining the right and wrong with cut-off points and flexibility range. These standards of morality along with normative and deviant behaviors are universal, because Islamic teachings are meant for whole world (Soskolne & Last, 2008).

In general, human beings regard laws as a way of upholding the values of society, but these laws must be based on religion.

The curriculum is formulated at a national level so it has the policy role for the medical education in Pakistan. Contemporary curriculum development is in place, but still a continuous revision process need to be effectively in place. The National Bioethics curriculum for undergraduate medical students is reviewed using the document review technique by the researcher. The curriculum is the part of MBBS curriculum developed by HEC and PMDC, Pakistan. The main sections of the curriculum involve the guiding principles, scheme of studies and details of courses for MBBS.

The curriculum specifies overlapping areas in more than one discipline like, genetics, bio-statistics, infectious diseases, diabetes mellitus, and ethics. But in the section of guiding principles 'Ethics' is specified as an additional subject to be taught, which is not made compulsory. The choice is to be made by the universities, implementing the curriculum. As the 'Ethics' curriculum is not specified as a separate subject, rather it is integrated in different disciplines. The curriculum aims at the application of knowledge and problem solving rather than only recall.

This curriculum available on the official web link of PMDC states, that the current curriculum is the first step towards developing a more comprehensive and detailed curriculum. The curriculum describes the need for integration between disciplines, but the decision of integration, how and to what extent, is mentioned as the responsibility of the university faculty. The curriculum stresses the need for developing desired humanistic attributes in a doctor with effective communication skills and good patient-doctor relationship. It is advised to the universities faculty, to devise methods that build these attributes among the students and test them. Yet the core curriculum for medical ethics varies from country to country and institution to institution. Core curricula on medical ethics are available (Doyal & Gillon, 1998).

The PMDC curriculum specifies the list of topics in bioethics in the Forensic Medicine discipline under the topic of "Laws in relation to medical men". In the document, the ethical and professional obligations of registered medical practitioner, towards Law and the PMDC are specified. The objectives of teaching ethics in Forensic Medicine includes; the development of doctor-patient relationship in the context of highest ethical standards, to understand and refrain from any temptations to professional misconduct, to guard professional secrets and privileged communication, to maintain highest ethical principles in medical examination and when obtaining consent and to define what constitutes medical negligence. In addition, to debate the pros and cons of organ transplantation in each individual case, to develop and defend a personal moral view on artificial insemination, therapeutic abortions, euthanasia, biomedical research etc. These learning outcomes are to be achieved, in keeping with the norms of society and highest ethical principles. The course content specified by PMDC curriculum, which is to be taught by Forensic Medicine needs to be elaborated giving the key competencies to be developed and the methodologies to be used for developing them, otherwise a lot of implementation issues will arise, as we currently experience in different medical colleges.

Medical Ethics core content, specified in the Community Medicine subject includes; background, concepts and components of medical ethics, along with national recommended guidelines and code of Medical Ethics. Medical Ethics content to be taught in clinical disciplines includes; effective communication with the patient, the family and the community regarding disease and its relevant issues, understand medical ethics and its application pertaining to surgery and maintain the confidentiality of the patient and provision of the opportunity to apply medical ethics' knowledge related to that field.

The PMDC curriculum mentions the Behavioral Sciences, as to be taught in Psychiatry. The curriculum document explains the desired outcome in a fresh medical graduate as; to have the knowledge and understanding of mechanism of body in health and disease along with knowledge of relevant behavior he has to show with patients, families and society; to have professional and communication skills to diagnose and manage diseases, to develop excellent communication skills with colleagues, doctors, nurses, paramedical staff and public and to have developed conditioned sympathetic attitude towards ailing humanity; Clinical Skills should have acquired by achieving a desired theoretical and practical level of competence according to the goals set up by the medical college. These outcomes can be achieved in Pakistani medical graduates, once the undergraduate students acquire the desired competence in medical ethics, by using core curriculum specified in the document under study, as well as, through hidden curriculum, which means the transmission of norms, values, and beliefs conveyed in both the formal educational content and the social interactions within these colleges. The role of "hidden curriculum" cannot be overlooked in medical ethics. A comprehensive ethics curriculum needs the understanding of broader cultural context, in the light of which the curriculum should be developed (Hafferty & Franks, 1994).

The medical ethics covers the practice ethics as well as the research ethics. A code of ethics is always there, to justify actions by individuals within a specific environment. The training of ethics, at undergraduate and post graduate level should be consistent and standardized, with unified depth and applying the principles which have reached a consensus of importance, using a consistent curriculum (Lakhan, Hamlat, McNamee & Laird, 2009). Community practices and processes are important as they are used to develop and critique learning and teaching approaches, policies and administration so the students and faculty develop ethical practices and professionalism.

The methodology generally mentioned in the PMDC curriculum includes many options, out of which a suitable methodology producing maximum output can be used. Problem-based Learning, Tutorials/Practical sessions/Essential Skills or Lab practice, clinical rotations and ward visits, Lectures/Seminars/CPC's - using modern audio-visual techniques, distant learning using electronic devices and current Information Technology facilities. Journal Club, Community -based learning and acquisition of Competencies through any other method can be used.

The PMDC curriculum contains only the objectives and course outline, but linking syllabus to the teaching or instructional and assessment methodology is inadequately explained. The suitable learning resources for undergraduates need to be specified. In addition, the time allocation for medical ethics training, strategies for implementation of the training in medical ethics and desired competencies development activities are not effectively addressed in the curriculum under review. The periodic or continuous assessment or examination of medical ethics course is not adequately mentioned. It is very difficult to assess students' competencies in medical ethics with out examining them and displaying their performance. The need for compulsory examination at undergraduate level to assess the ability of medical students to reason critically and logically on ethical issues cannot be denied (Boyd, 1987). If there is no formal assessment in ethics, this downgrade the course and leads to its being classified as optional, either officially or at least in the perception of students. This results in poor attendance and uncertain acquisition of ethical skills (Calman & Downie, 1987).

The detailed content required for medical ethics competency development should be developed by involving local stakeholders like, medical educationists, ethicists and experienced faculty in medical schools, colleges and universities. A strong forum can be used, as in Pakistan's case the Higher Education Commission of Pakistan is the umbrella body and Pakistan Medical and Dental Council is the platform for; policy formulation, curricular planning, designing, implementing, evaluating and reviewing the curricula in medical ethics education. The policy transfer concept can also be utilized as a curricular transfer from medical universities and schools; where continuous, meticulous research has been done developing the curricula. The transfer or adaptation is conditioned with the incorporation of and modifications according to context specific needs, demands, priorities, and resources along with considering the socio-cultural, economic, religious and political forces in Pakistan.

The use of developed and tested curricula for teaching at undergraduate level; has been practiced but the efforts fail when it is not context specific. The environment where the young medical graduate is going to work and practice is the defining and determining force for ethical practice. In Pakistan, the society and community, where the young doctors practice, consist of divergent healthcare setups including, allopath, homeopath, Hikmat, Chinese medicine and other indigenous health practices like Unani- medicine etc. In addition to these the "Quacks/traditional healers" play their role by practicing medicine in our streets. Majority of our population is dependent on these practitioners and have a good faith in them.

The curriculum change through review and context specific insight is needed for the medical ethics curriculum used at national level in Pakistan. An unethical practice, by untrained physicians, non-physician practitioners, indigenous health care practitioners and quacks (An untrained person who pretends to be a physician and dispenses medical advice and treatment) is a threat for medical professionalism. The document on Human Resources for Health (Joint Learning Initiative, 2004) and World Health Report (World Health Organization, 2006) estimated a huge gap in availability and demand of trained health human resource. It means major portion of Pakistani population is depending on health care providers, which are inadequately trained in ethical practices and professionalism as the curriculum used at national level inadequately addresses the competencies in medical ethics.

In Pakistan, the current curriculum needs change by incorporating more structured, ethics based, integrated training of medical undergraduates. We need to produce 'community friendly health care providers', which will work at grass root level, in the community in a more friendly and professional way. The responsibilities of medical universities and the medical colleges in Pakistan are much more in the implementation of the curriculum in its full spirit. As there are private sector medical colleges, emerging in medical education in Pakistan, it is becoming difficult and tedious task to bring them in the streamline, where they can implement bioethics education for medical students uniformly and produce graduates with same competency level in medical ethics.

After the review of the medical ethics curriculum used at national level, the next objective was to assess the need for change in the curriculum and to determine the nature of change required, through in-depth interviews, author's insight and analysis. Analysis identifies the areas and nature of change required, as; making the curriculum of medical ethics compulsory for undergraduate medical teaching and training, bridging the gaps in ethics core content written in curriculum, elaborating and specifying the resources required for ethics teaching in the curriculum, specifying teaching, training and assessment methodologies in the curriculum. Other important points emerged from the analysis are; to create awareness among the stakeholders, about the need for inculcating medical ethics in medical students and training of the faculty in medical ethics.

Medical Ethics is not considered as a separate subject in PMDC curriculum which creates difficulty in sensitizing the faculty, about the changing trends in medical ethics education. The implementation of curricular change demands the establishment of Medical Ethics & Behavioral Sciences Department in every medical college. To make curriculum ethics friendly, we need to incorporate more comprehensive and structured training component on medical ethics. Medical ethics teaching and training should be done throughout the five year medical program and it should be mandatory for the affiliated medical universities to design comprehensive pan for the implementation of medical ethics curriculum. Throughout the teaching program of undergraduate studies the formative and summative assessment of knowledge and competencies need to be done. All these changes require structured reforms in undergraduate medical ethics curriculum, focusing on developing more integrated and learner-centered curriculum.

Focusing on the curricular reforms in Medical Ethics, we need to understand the context of Pakistan, where it is to be implemented. Contemporary curriculum change process must be based on principles, like; ensuring quality, relevance to the need and context, and involving a range of stakeholders. Common topics that need to be incorporated in the content of medical ethics curriculum are; professionalism, ethics codes and oaths, paternalism, competency, truthfulness, confidentiality, informed consent, abortion, maternal-fetal issues, end-of-life decisions, decisions on death and dying, physician-assisted suicide, research on human subjects, treatment for incompetent patients, objectivity and bias in medical research, issues in protection of human subjects, animal research issues, genetic testing, managed care, health care reform, social justice and health care, organ donation and procurement, health care regulation, ethics committees, medical futility, unfair aspects of the health care system, and pain control etc. In later years of training in medical colleges additional teaching and training about moral, professional, and legal obligations of physicians, physicians' traditions and responsibilities in developing and implementing health care delivery etc. must be incorporated.

These topics must be discussed, analyzed and students should be encouraged to give their opinions and reasoning. Curriculum must have the option of electives in Medical Ethics and Humanities. The competencies required to be addressed in Medical Ethics curriculum are; to develop skills for critical evaluation and articulation of moral and philosophical claims, arguments, and goals in medical practice and medical literature, to formulate, present, and defend a particular position on a moral or policy issue in health care, to be able to communicate these ideas and conclusions effectively, to patients, patients' families, colleagues and other decision makers in society, both orally and in writing, and to reflect on the relationships in moral, professional, and legal obligations of physicians, including those involving honesty, and respect for patient well-being, autonomy, dignity and confidentiality (Department of Medical Humanities, n.d.).

Grading in these courses should be based on written and oral exams, class participation, short papers, and case presentations. Ethics learning among students occur passively, by apprenticeship mode of medical education. We can mention in the curriculum about the use didactic lectures, small group discussions, standardized patients, ethics rounds etc. to improve students' learning. It is general consensus by most bio-ethicists that realistic case based discussions are the best methodology of imparting bioethics education (Christakis & Feudtner, 1993). Now-a-days, content of core competencies are developing as a part of the subject curriculum.

Teachers, who are in contact with medical students from pre-clinical days onwards, to the time of internships, electives and house jobs, impart their ethical views by creating an example, becoming a role model and by precept, but such passive learning by 'osmosis' is insufficient. Knowledge base must be imparted in order to enrich the student with in depth understanding of ethical judgments on clinical problems during the undergraduate years. The learning process continues even after graduation and it evolves with maturity and experience. The willingness of the teacher to debate and discuss ethical issues is very important for student learning (Bicknell, 1985).

Development of medical ethics education is spread over history (Goldie, 2000). The content of undergraduate medical ethics education is the area on which consensus develops easily, but selection and development of appropriate teaching and assessment methods are difficult areas. Barriers to the successful implementation of the core curriculum in medical ethics in Pakistan are; unavailability of appropriate resources and academic expertise, poor curriculum integration both horizontally as well as vertically and poor consolidation of learning, the choice and use of inappropriate assessment methods. One important aspect is the human resource for teaching and training in medical ethics. For this purpose research showed that an interdisciplinary group of teachers is much effective (Fox, Arnold & Brody, 1995). Variation in the content of teaching of medical ethics exists from institution to institution and region to region (DuBois & Burkemper, 2000). The need to have a uniform curriculum is growing very fast.

In Pakistan, medical ethics curriculum for undergraduates needs to be revised and rebuilt by developing frameworks for the change process and using them for successful implementation of the change. Content of core competencies can be developed by utilizing services of Ethicists and educationists or can be adopted from institutions serving in medical ethics. Frameworks showing curriculum change process are given as, Figure 1 and 2. These frameworks show the pathway towards change and the areas of change in medical ethics curriculum in Pakistan. Curriculum change is a dynamic process aimed at ensuring the relevance of learning (UNESCO, n.d.). Due to the changing demands of patients, practice, and society the Medical Education is continually facing problems in student learning especially in medical ethics. Reforms are required to bring a real productive change. Strategic management literature shows that content is one of the three elements essential for successful change, which are content, context, and the change process. The relationship between them is very important. (Savage, 2011).

In Canada, a shared curriculum framework was developed which support the design, delivery and evaluation of global health curriculum. (Redwood-Campbell, Pakes, Rouleau, MacDonald, Arya, Purkey, et al. 2011). The frameworks developed show the need for a context specific but unified core curriculum for the globe. There is growing demand of medical ethicists to teach. They will be best suited to teach medical students. They have first hand experience of common ethical issues and a good knowledge base of ethics, to be able to deal with the real problems faced in the clinical environment by the students. The need for improving the medical ethics curriculum in Pakistani medical schools is unquestionable. Trained human resource is required, which can develop and implement a culturally and regionally relevant medical ethics curriculum at national level and get it included in medical education curriculum of Pakistan (Jafarey, 2003). Fostering, developing and managing curriculum change is dynamic process. Context specific instructional and assessment methodology shift is required.

A paper by Hyder, Merritt, Ali, Tran, Subramaniamb & Akhtar (2008) seeks to describe the ethics processes in play when public-health mechanisms are established in low- and middle-income countries. This shows the importance of ethics education for practitioners and at an institutional level. The assessment methodologies should be inline with the objectives of the program or the learning outcomes developed, primarily aimed at determining the quality of the students' ethics knowledge base. This paper by Mitchell, Myser & Kerridge, (1993) describes the strengths and limitations of a purely knowledge based method of evaluation and also the redefining the assessment in ethics. The term, 'clinical ethical competency' is used for the actual application of knowledge by the students in a controlled clinical context.

The framework for the change in curriculum is developed using the contextual information of Pakistani undergraduate medical education curriculum (Figure 1). Pakistan's cultural, religious, ethical, social, economic and geo-political context is unique, having its own ethical issues, taboos, myths, lifestyle and mind set. In such diverse situation; the need for context specific curriculum for medical ethics teaching and training of undergraduate medical students is of crucial importance. Written and hidden curriculum, both are important and must be addressed while implementing the ethics curriculum. The medical professional ethics also include the ethics while dealing with patients, their relatives and attendants, along with ethical issues in their professional relationship with their colleagues or the health care team members (including doctors, nurses, paramedics and support staff). The curriculum should address how to discuss and manage those issues? The other area in medial ethics is the health research ethics which need to be given much attention in this curriculum, as it has not been addressed formally for the undergraduates.

In the curricular change framework, health research ethics are incorporated, so the students are trained using real research studies in which they can identify major and minor ethical issues, address them and also understand the role of Institutional Review Boards and the need for their ethical clearance for protection of each and every human subject's right. They can get a better understanding of plagiarism and other ethical issues in research.

The framework also covers the ethics in Public Health, targeting individuals in families and communities. Ethical issues in Public Health practice are important to teach as the students are going to work at grass root level in primary health care centers, where they have to deal with real world ethical cases, issues and situations. Sound knowledge base along with training using ethical case studies can help improve the ethical practices of doctors.

The ethical principles are the foundation of a personality so the medical ethics teaching should start from first year, spreading up to final year and even more practical training for interns and post graduates. Development of curricular content in specific contextual environment is required. A range of instructional and appropriate assessment methodologies should be given, so the universities can make their own choice; achieving maximum learning outcomes. The competencies must be developed in medical ethics and the disciplines involved in accomplishing the objectives of achieving these competencies must be clearly specified. Assessment should be scheduled throughout the five years study duration, which will make medical ethics a cross-cutting discipline. Ethicists or faculty trained in medical ethics should run the department of medical ethics and run the teaching programs.

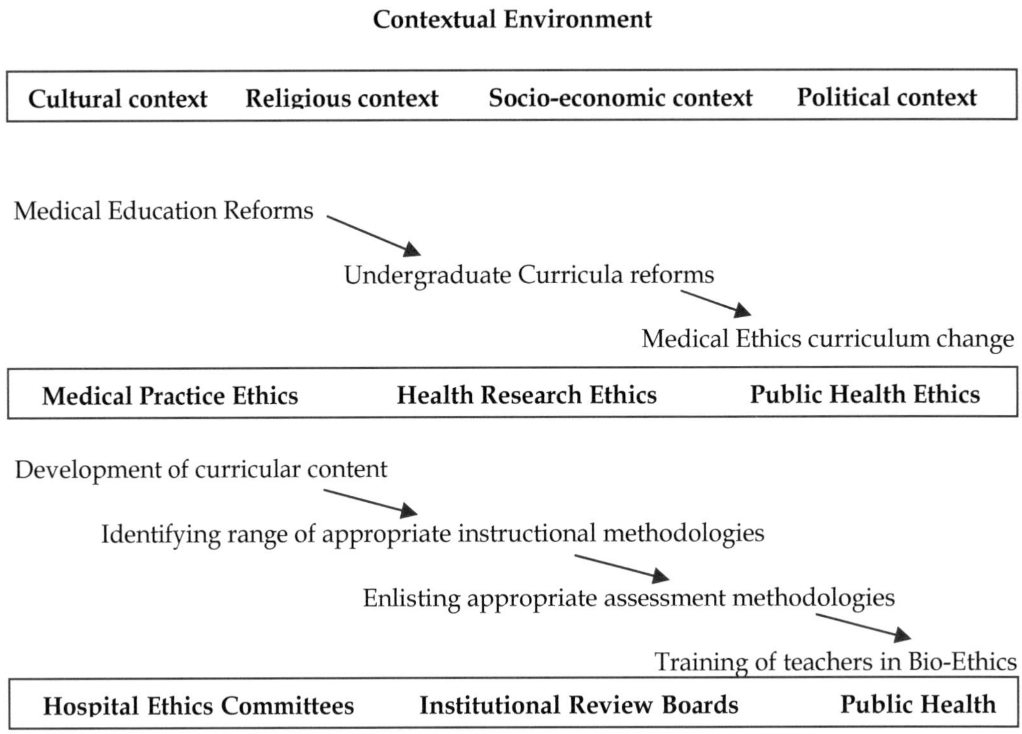
Contextual Environment
Cultural context
Religious context
Socio-economic context
Political context
Medical Education Reforms
Undergraduate Curricula reforms
Medical Ethics curriculum change
Medical Practice Ethics
Health Research Ethics
Public Health Ethics
Development of curricular content
Identifying range of appropriate instructional methodologies
Enlisting appropriate assessment methodologies
Training of teachers in Bio-Ethics
Hospital Ethics Committees
Institutional Review Boards
Public Health

Fig. 1. Framework for Curricular change process

Curricular change will be more sustainable and productive if based on reforms in medical education, including more structured training in medical ethics throughout the medical training at undergraduate as well as post graduate levels. The change process will be slow and requiring more professional attitude of policy makers, medical educationists, ethicists and teachers. The ethics teaching starts from the cradle in form of moral values shapes under the influence of religion, culture, social, economic and political environment. The teachers play a very crucial role in teaching basic and professional ethics after parents. Teachers acting as mentors facilitate the learning of students by acting as role models for them.

Medical ethicists face more responsibility than other teachers to become mentors and developing their mentoring skills for improving and facilitating student learning in medical ethics. Teaching medical ethics is not to create Medical Ethicists but to equip the medical doctors with competency to identify ethical issues and dilemmas which they can come across in their medical practice, perform ethical analysis and make judicious decisions; using the knowledge and experience gained from their training at undergraduate level.

Medical Education Curricular reforms for undergraduates will cover the area of medical ethics. The need for reforms can be assessed by reviewing the curriculum available and comparing it with the globally adapted curricula, the expected qualities of a medical graduate, through survey based assessment of the quality of ethics teaching in medical schools and students' satisfaction with the current teaching program on medical ethics. Reforms will bring uniformity in the curricula and their implementation and evaluation strategies in Pakistan. The Curricular change process will involve, specifying the areas of change, duration of change process, time frame for change, feed back on change, strategies for implementation of change and monitoring of change process in medical universities and schools. The principles for the change will be, the adult learning (Pedagogy), educational context and knowledge base. The change should be learner centered, integrated into other disciplines, competency based and assessment oriented.

The change process should be working strategically not randomly and under the umbrella of reforms. Curriculum is every thing we do and use of emerging technology, and diversity in it can make curricular change a continuous process. The entire curricular change will be meaningless without the feed back system, so it should be in-built. Informed decision making is essential for deciding reforms and implementing change. The depth, horizontal integration and vertical spreading of the curriculum need to be focused while developing it.

Figure 2, shows the framework for the implementation of curricular change. It explains the type of curriculum which could be used, the course for which it is applied, the areas covered, target population, disciplines involved, outcome desired/ qualities in a graduate, appropriate instructional methodologies and assessment of competencies and knowledge. The framework will help the medical educationists in curriculum planning and development in Pakistan's context.

The instructional methods used world over are tested and proven to be effective in promoting students' learning. Still more research is required on developing and testing instructional and assessment methodologies. Case scenarios and real case studies along with mock case discussions help a lot in students' learning. The students are made ethically sensitive, with motivation for solving ethical dilemmas. Their mind set is positively changed through mentorship for enhancing their skills and competencies for ethical analysis, reasoning and judicial judgments in real situations especially in doctor-patient and doctor-doctor relationships.

Teaching methods traditionally used for promoting ethical thinking and 'moral reasoning' for undergraduates and postgraduates have included lectures, ethics case conferences, discussions of films and other techniques (Strong, Connelly & Forrow, 1992). Many studies are available to share the experience of appropriate methodology use in medical ethics education. Small group discussions help the learning through detailed discussion on managing the ethical dilemma by facilitating the capabilities of students for ethical reasoning and analyzing the situation through empathy.

Curriculum	Target course	Ethics areas	Whom to deal with	Disciplines involved	Desired outcomes	Appropriate instructional methodology	Assessment of ethical knowledge and competence
Written curriculum Hidden curriculum	Under graduate medical students	-Professional Ethics/Medical Practice Ethics -Health Research Ethics -Public Health Ethics	-Patients -Attendants/ relatives -Health care team members (Doctors, nurses, paramedics) -Human subjects -Individuals in the families and communities	Teaching and training by; -Forensic Medicine -Community Medicine -Behavioral sciences -Every clinical specialty involved	-Positive attitude -Effective communication -Empathy -Taking informed consent -Keeping confidentiality -Keeping privacy -Respect for patients' rights -Doing no harm -Working in interest of the subject/ patient -Doing fairness and equality (justice) -Truthfulness and honesty -Ability to conduct Ethical analysis of cases -Ability to give ethical reasoning	-Assigning and discussing Case studies -Using Mock Case scenarios -Lectures -Seminars -Problem based learning	-Multiple choice questions -Ethical analysis and reasoning on given cases in oral examination -Objectively Structured Clinical Examination

Fig. 2. Frame work for curricular change implementation

In Pakistan's context, the curriculum used uniformly throughout the public and private sector medical education institutions, is given by PMDC which is responsible for laying down the guidelines for medical education and curricula development. Our misfortune is that our curricula are not flexible to adapt changes occurring globally. The change or review process is slow and leading to 'educational obsolescence'. We are not moving at the same pace as of the world renowned medical education institutions. Due to globalization it is dire need of today, that Pakistan make medical education reforms and use more comprehensive, integrated and learner centered curricula and implement it throughout the medical institutions.

A high degree of faulty motivation is required and must be achieved before initiating the curricular change process. The motivated faculty will participate in informed decision making, for the curricular change process; in addition, they will enable transition from the current curriculum to the integrated, learner centered curriculum much smooth and easier during the implementation process. Faculty training is very essential in Pakistan's context. The in-service training of faculty about the changing demands of undergraduate medical education in the field of bioethics is essential.

Bioethics education has gained its importance in Pakistan. A large number of organizations are working for it, at postgraduate level and for practicing health care providers, including doctors, nurses, paramedics etc. Many organizations are providing recognized training in Bioethics. At the undergraduate level as PMDC is the only authority to develop curricula so what ever is given in it is implemented with exceptions in few medical teaching institute in private sector. It is a tedious process but if we start right now, we can enter the main stream of changing medical education trends. The political will and commitment at national level will be the determining and driving force for curricular reforms in medical education. This will bring our graduates at power with the developed world professionals.

The summary of all the discussions done in this chapter, by using the document review technique, in-depth interviews, literature review and author's analysis; highlights the need for curricular change in the field of medical ethics. The proposed frameworks show, the areas in medical ethics curriculum that need context specific change and modification, using state of the art methodologies.

2. References

Batool, Z., Qureshi, R. H. Quality Assurance Manual for higher education In Pakistan Higher education commission. Retrieved from, http://qa.nust.edu.pk/downloads/Quality_Assurance_Manual.pdf

Battat, R., Seidman, G., Chadi, N., Chanda, M.Y., Nehme, J., Hulme, J., Li, A., Faridi, N., & Brewer, T. F. (2010). Global health competencies and approaches in medical education: a literature review. *BMC Medical Education*, 10, 94. PubMed Central Full Text

Bicknell, D. J. (1985). Current arrangements for teaching medical ethics to undergraduate medical students. *Journal of medical ethics, 11*, 25-26 Retrieved from, www.ncbi.nlm.nih.gov/pmc/articles/.../pdf/jmedeth00252-0029.pdf

Bobbitt, Franklin, J. (1918). *The Curriculum.* Boston: Houghton Mifflin.

Boyd, W., & Newton, D. (2011). Times of Change, Times of Turbulence: Seeking an Ethical Framework for Curriculum Development during Critical Transition in Higher Education. *International Journal of Cyber Ethics in Education (IJCEE),* 1 (3), 11. Retrieved from, http://www.igi-global.com/article/international-journal-cyber-ethics-education/56104

Boyd, K. M. (1987). Report of a working party on the teaching of medical ethics - The Pond report. London: IME Publications.

Calman, K. C., Downie, R. S. (1987). Practical problems in the teaching of ethics to medical students. *Journal of medical ethics, 13,* 153-156

Christakis, D. A., & Feudtner, C. (1993). Ethics in a short white coat: the ethical dilemmas that medical students confront. *Acad Med, 68,* 249-54.

Coles, C. (2003). 'The development of a curriculum for spinal surgeons', Observations following the Second Spine Course of the Spinal Society of Europe Barcelona. Retrieved from, http://www.eurospine.org/Teachers%20Course/C_Coles_report_03.html,

Department of Medical Humanities. Medical ethics Curriculum. Retrieved from, http://www.ecu.edu/cs-dhs/medhum/medEthicsCurriculum.cfm

Doyal, L., Gillon, R. (May 30, 1998). Medical ethics and law as a core subject in medical education, Editorial. *BMJ,* 316, 1623. Retrieved from, http://www.bmj.com/content/316/7145/1623.full

DuBois, J. M., & Burkemper, J. (2000). Ethics education in US medical schools: a study of syllabi. *Acad Med, 77,* 432-37.

EduQnA.com (2007). What is the meaning of curriculum? and what are the examples of curriculum? Retrieved from, http://www.eduqna.com/Other/175-other.html.

Evans, M., Greaves, D. (2001). 'Developing the medical humanities'–report of a research colloquium, and collected abstracts of papers. *Med Humanities,(27),* 93-98 doi:10.1136/mh.27.2.93

Fox, E., Arnold, R. M., & Brody, B. (1995). Medical ethics education: Past Present and Future. *Acad Med, 70,* 761-68.

Goldie, J. (2000). Review of ethics curricula in undergraduate medical education. *Medical Education, 34,* 108–119. doi: 10.1046/j.1365-2923.2000.00607.x

Government of Pakistan (September 11, 2002). Ordinance No.LIII of 2002.

Hafferty, F. W., Franks, R. (November, 1994). The hidden curriculum, ethics teaching, and the structure of medical education. *Acad Med., 69* (11), 861-71.

Harvard School of Public Health. (n.d.). Global Research Ethics Map – https://webapps.sph.harvard.edu/live/gremap/view.cfm?country=Pakistan

Higher Education Commission of Pakistan. (2002). Curriculum Revision. http://www.hec.gov.pk/INSIDEHEC/DIVISIONS/AECA/CURRICULUMREVISION/Pages/CurriculumRevision.aspx

Hyder, A. A., Merritt, M., Ali, J., Tran, N. T., Subramaniamb, K. & Akhtar, T. (2008). Integrating ethics, health policy and health systems in low- and middle-income countries: case studies from Malaysia and Pakistan. *Bulletin of the World Health Organization, 86,* 606–611. Retrieved from, http://www.who.int/bulletin/volumes/86/8/08-051110.pdf

Redwood-Campbell, L., Pakes, B., Rouleau, K., MacDonald, C., J., Arya, N., Purkey, E.,et.al. (2011). Developing a curriculum framework for global health in family medicine:

emerging principles, competencies, and educational approaches. *BMC Medical Education*, 11, 46. doi:10.1186/1472-6920-11-46

Jafarey, A. M. (2003). Bioethics and Medical Education, *JMPA, 53* (6). Retrieved from, http://jpma.org.pk/full_article_text.php?article_id=160

Joint Learning Initiative (2004). Human Resources for Health: overcoming the Crisis. Cambridge: Harvard University Press.

Kimmelman, J., Weijer, C., Meslin, E. (2009). "Helsinki discords: FDA, ethics, and international drug trials". *The Lancet, 373* (9657), 13–4. doi:10.1016/S0140-6736(08)61936-4.

Lakhan, S.E., Hamlat, E., McNamee, T., Laird, C. (2009). "Time for a unified approach to medical ethics". *Philosophy, Ethics, and Humanities in Medicine, 4* (3), 13. doi:10.1186/1747-5341-4-13.

McCrary, S. V. (April 2001). The Role of Bioethics in Medical Education: A Crucial Profession Under Threat. ActionBioscience.org. Retrieved from, http://www.actionbioscience.org/biotech/mccrary.html

Mitchell, K. R., Myser, C., & Kerridge, I. H. (December, 1993). Assessing the clinical ethical competence of undergraduate medical students. *J Med Ethics, 9* (4): 230–236. Retrieved from, http://www.ncbi.nlm.nih.gov/pmc/articles/PMC1376346/

Pakistan Medical and Dental Council. (n.d.) http://www.pmrc.org.pk/nbc.htm

Pakistan Medical and Dental Council. (n.d.)Code of Ethics. http://www.pmdc.org.pk/ethics.htm

Pakistan Medical & Dental Council & Higher Education Commission Islamabad (2005). Curriculum for M.B.B.S. Retrieved from, http://dev.plexushosting.com/pmdc/LinkClick.aspx?fileticket=EKfBIOSDTkE%3d&tabid=102&mid=556

Pakistan Medical and Dental Council (June 5, 1962). Ordinance. http://dev.plexushosting.com/pmdc/LinkClick.aspx?fileticket=7AY1%2fco4suQ%3d&tabid=102&mid=588

Savage, C. (2011). Overcoming Inertia in Medical Education: Navigating Change with Adaptive Reflection (Doctoral dissertation, Karolinska Institutet, 2011). http://hdl.handle.net/10616/40606)
http://ki.academia.edu/CarlSavage/Papers/730900/Overcoming_Inertia_in_Medical_Education_Navigating_Change_with_Adaptive_Reflection

Soskolne, C. L. & Last, J. M. (2008). Ethics and Public Health Policy. In Wallace, R. B. (Ed.), *Public Health and Preventive Medicine* (15th edition.), (pp. 27-37). USA:MacGraw-Hill.

Strong, C., Connelly, J. E. & Forrow, L. (1992). Teachers' perceptions of difficulties in teaching ethics in residences. *Academic medicine, 67*, 398-402.

UNESCO. (2003). Ethics Education Programme. Retrieved from, http://www.unesco.org/new/en/social-and-human-sciences/themes/ethics-education-programme/

UNESCO. (n.d.) http://www.ibe.unesco.org/fileadmin/user_upload/archive/publications/regworkshops/finrep_pdf/wsrep_philippines_06.pdf

UNESCO. (n.d.)The Worldwide Resource Pack in Curriculum Change - Overview http://www.ibe.unesco.org/fileadmin/user_upload/COPs/Pages_documents/Resource_Packs/WWRP_Overview.pdf

U.S. National Institutes of Health, Office of Human Subjects Research. "Nuremberg Code". Retrieved on November 17, 2011, http://ohsr.od.nih.gov/guidelines/nuremberg.html.

Wojtczak, A. (2002). Glossary of Medical Education Terms. Retrieved from, http://www.iime.org/glossary.htm.

World Health Organization (2006). World Health Report 2006: Working together for Health. Geneva: WHO.

Zaidi, S. A. (1987). Undergraduate medical education in underdeveloped countries: the case of Pakistan. *Soc Sci Med, 25* (8), 911-9. [Abstract] Retrieved from, http://www.ncbi.nlm.nih.gov/pubmed/3317891

9

Medical Ethics in the Czech Republic – Experiences in the Post-Totalitarian Country

Jiri Simek[1], Eva Krizova[2] and Lenka Zamykalova[1]
[1]*South Bohemian University in Ceske Budejovice*
[2]*Technical University of Liberec -Institute of Health Studies*
Czech Republic

1. Introduction

Countries in Central Europe undergo various transformations in society and economics; interpersonal relationships change, and new civic and political structures emerge. All changes take place in a relatively short period, and they are directed to establish the same organisation of public affairs that is common in Western Europe. For this reason we can also see these countries as a natural sociology laboratory; ongoing processes are more transparent and some universally accepted theses could be re-examined.

Bohemia has been an integral part of Europe for centuries, and was therefore culturally tightly bound with other European countries. For fifty years its European identity (1939 - 1989) was interrupted by totalitarian regimes, of which the Communist regime was the most influential; it lasted from 1948 till 1989. Communist ideology was egalitarian and intentionally preferred society to individuals, therefore the Communist regime was characterised by strong paternalism of political and state administration. The Czech society is traditionally quite egalitarian with strong aversion against big social differences. These tendencies were strengthened by the Communist regime in its underlying egalitarian theory. Some positive human rights, such as a right to health care, to a job, and to housing, were fairly met. Social security was on a high level. The price for this was almost a complete lack of civil liberties. Basic civil rights, such as a right to free speech, to free association, and to free movement were abolished. In the paternalistic, ideologically driven regime not only civil but also working initiative markedly declined. The well known result was economic retardation, worsening of the environment, and life expectancy also stagnated. Due to the absence of civil liberties all the negative effects were kept secret.

From an ethical point of view the most devastating effects of this regime was the breakdown of public debate and the disregard for language. Public debate is no simple enterprise; it must be practiced in the society, and be adapted to the changing social and technical conditions of each generation. In the second half of twentieth century citizens in Western countries were more and more forced to negotiate in politics, civil communities, at offices, and in health care. Thanks to this necessity they gained good skills in negotiation. In countries with a Communist totalitarian regime arguments were of no use; what was much more important was favour of powerful politicians and later on also a position in informal exchange of scarce services and goods. Public debate was systematically suppressed, causing people in post-communist countries to lack skills in everyday negotiations. They even lacked an awareness of the necessity of negotiation, and the capability to negotiate. For example, the political scene has been seriously polarised in past years. There are no visible attempts to make political agreements across the political spectrum. In the latest elections (June 2010) voters showed their strong dissatisfaction, and the traditionally strongest parties lost. Two entirely new parties entered the Parliament and created a government with a weak right wing party. In some areas the parties' programs distinctly differ, but in the realistic understanding that the trust of voters could be easily lost, the three parties manage to negotiate solutions acceptable to all of them. Only rarely are their competencies in negotiation acknowledged in the media.

After 1989 the Czech Republic changed its political regime in a very short time, and became a country in transition from totalitarian to democratic. Restoration of democratic institutions was quite a simple task, since there was a history of its existence, at least in the interwar period 1918-1939. Also the nongovernmental sector has boomed rapidly, and the stakeholders of civil society began to actively influence political and social life. The most difficult part was the restoration of civil thought, the interioration of civil values, cultivation of political culture, and the practice of public debate, though it is constantly improving. (Simek, 1999)

Between 1948 and 1952 the centralized tax funded health care system was introduced in Czechoslovakia to replace the Bismarckian mix of mandatory and private health insurance. As in other socialist countries, a universal access to health care free of charge in the place of use was guaranteed. A hierarchical structure of primary, secondary, and tertiary health care was built up, and stipulated areas of geographical accessibility existed for users. Physicians became state employees and private medical care became illegal. Due to poor outcomes on the population's health status, the socialist health care system became the subject of critical remarks already in the perestroika period (mid 1980´s). This resulted in a very urgent need for a health care system transformation immediately after the Velvet Revolution. A new system was outlined, which re-established the public health insurance, mandatory for all citizens in Czechoslovakia, and from 1993 in the Czech and Slovak Republic, which had split. Provision of ambulatory care was completely privatised, although still financed from public health insurance. A large number of regional hospitals was also privatised, so a mix of state-run, regional/municipal, and private hospitals participated in-patient services. In a very short period, the status of providers changed from the employee in the public services towards a free-lance professional or entrepreneur. Values of personal responsibility for health, which have compensated for the unlimited solidarity, were manifested in patients' co-payments for drugs, certain services, consumer's fees, etc. Positively, during the health care transformation a massive technological modernization and availability of foreign drugs led to a steep improvement in the quality of medical care. Simultaneously, attention was also paid to ethical issues and to psychological and moral issues.

1.1 Medical ethics as a discipline – Theory and practice

During socialism medical ethics did not exist as a separate discipline, though the term was often used in the debate on medical practice. The Marxist-Leninist ideology was considered be a sufficient philosophical foundation and reservoir of advices for medical doctors. Due to the restriction of civil liberties, medical professionals had evolved into a highly paternalistic mode of behaviour to the patient. Patients had very limited freedom of choice of the provider, and no means to control the outcomes of clinical practice. However, it would be too simplistic to depict the practice in black and white colours, since the practice was always diverse although a few responsive and paternalistic patterns have culturally dominated. During the socialist period the deontological approach stressed the medical duties instead of patients' rights. Naturally, one of the consequences of the Velvet Revolution in 1989 was a strict demand to humanize the medical practice and eliminate the patients' submissiveness. In 1992, The Charter of Patients' Rights was adopted by the Ethics Committee of the Ministry of Health and in 2001. The Convention on Human Rights and Bioethics of the Council of Europe was approved by the Czech Parliament, which implied radical legal amendments to enhance legal patients' rights.

Medical ethics as an academic discipline started to develop early after the change of the regime. Universities regained their academic freedoms, and study programs were modernised. Medical ethics issues were implemented in all health care programs. In 1990 chairs or institutes specialised in medical ethics were founded in 4 schools of medicine. In this way an institutional base was established. Important aid came from abroad, mostly in the form of donations of books and libraries. The most important help came from the American "The Hastings Centre." The founder and president of The Hastings Centre, Daniel Callahan, created an Eastern European Program, and dozens of people from post-communist countries were invited to The Hastings Centre for the six-week study stay. Later on Daniel Callahan visited Prague many times; he gave lectures, and helped with the organisation of seminars and conferences. In 2008 he received a doctorate honoris causa at the Charles University in Prague. At this time medical or health care ethics were taught at all schools educating future physicians and non-medical health care professionals. Some research was also developed in the Czech Republic. Further development of medical ethics faced two difficulties: the lack of interest of the public in ethics in general, and the lack of an institutional background outside medical schools. There is no chair for ethics at schools of philosophy in the Czech Republic.

The following texts are a summary of the results of our research done in 1999 - 2009 in four consecutive projects funded by the Grant Agency of the Czech Republic. We put together information, which we just published in relevant journals. (Krizova & Simek, 2002; Krizova & Simek, 2007; Simek at el. 2009; Simek et al. 2010) In the research we have addressed three issues that we use as case examples of how medical ethics in the Czech Republic has manifested in the debate, and how it was implemented in everyday practice.

2. Informed consent in the CR

As we have already mentioned above, a discrepancy existed between legal norms and practice during socialism. The Law No. 20/1966 Coll., "On the Care for the People's Health ", has vaguely stated the physicians' duty to inform the sick, but it was the physician who could decide whether and how much information he/she will communicate.

The communication between physicians and patients was identified as a significant problem already in early nineties. "Medicine of secrecy" was identified as the biggest fault of the system (Haškovcová, 2002) and truthfulness was considered to be an important value. Since then big progress was made and we can say that the Czech health care has definitely abandoned "medicine of secrecy." In this way the most active and progressive of all were paediatricians and oncologists, but also other specialists and general practitioners who began to extensively and consequently inform their patients. At university hospitals informed consent was introduced mainly thanks to regular contacts with Western European physicians and it was used as a way to document patient's consent with more invasive examination and therapy procedures. Since about 2002 informed consent was slowly introduced also in smaller and rural hospitals. (Zamykalová & Šimek, 2007) There were two impulses for its introduction. The first incentive was the start of the accreditation processes of Czech hospitals; implementation of informed consent in the clinical work was an essential part of accreditation requirements. The second, more important but later impulse was the approval of the European Convention on Human Rights and Biomedicine by the Czech Parliament in 2001, which resulted in amendments in the Czech health care legislation. In 2007 the Ministerial Decree No. 64/2007 on health care documentation was approved, and the legal provision of informed consent is the part of this Decree. Informed consent was also embedded in the Law on the Care for the People's Health.

Surprisingly, shared decision making was not the issue at that time. Implementation of informed consent is an example of a "reversed" process in the development of rules. Regulatory and legal measures recommended by the EU were first accepted, and then their meaning and sense were discussed. The dominant issues in the debate are formal aspects of informed consent -the length of texts, their content, and their storage in charts, which therapeutic and diagnostic procedures are subjects of this provision. Interest in the lay public is quite low; discussants are mainly health care providers. They tend to understand informed consent as a tool for protecting physicians from patient's complaints and law suits. Sometimes informed consent is submitted to patients as a merely formal affair and patients sign it without any further explanation during the admission process in the hospital.

The low interest of the public in informed consent was confirmed in our interviews with physicians, nurses and patients. Very often, the communication is short, sometimes patients do not have the opportunity to discuss all details and inquire about therapeutic options, risks, and benefits. On the other hand, Czech physicians quite often complained that patients were not interested in medical information which they tried to give them. In the research interviews patients expressed their wish to have conversation with their physicians but they did not seek information first. Instead, patients searched for the interest of physicians in their case, preferably personal interest and not only in their body and disease. They also wanted to be calmed down. The majority of patients understood the signature of informed consent sheet as a mere formal procedure. In a survey conducted in 2004 (1619 adults) only 42% of the population has correctly comprehended both aspects of the concept of the informed consent - right to information and right to approve/refuse the intervention. 31% of respondents admitted that they did not understand the term at all.

From the very beginning some physicians tried to give the patients a form of general consent with the treatment without the procedures being specified. This approach was immediately criticised by health lawyers and later on abandoned. In spite of this, 65% of respondents in our survey answered positively (definitely yes or probably yes) to this question: "I consent to the performance of an operation of the kind and of the extent that the surgeon shall decide according to the need that emerges during the operation." Do you find this kind of formulation acceptable? (Krizova & Simek, 2007)

Even though the situation has significantly improved, insufficient practice in how informed consent is carried out persists. The patients' age and education also affect the attitudes. Less educated and older patients still represent the passive position, whereas the younger and better educated users demand on more information and are more active in the decision process. Younger physicians also consider the informed consent as an appropriate demand of the sick. Despite the fact that much has been improved, some negative effects still prevail since informed consent is often deemed as the means of legal protection for the provider (physician, hospital) and less as a means of self-determination of the patient.

In Czech health care family members are quite often better informed than the patients themselves, and patients mostly agree with this practice. Maybe it overcomes some difficulties in communicating serious information. The family member translates the physicians' wording into the family's common language. On the contrary to physicians, family members recognize individual goals of their neighbours and honour their preferences in values. In this context, "shared decision making" takes place within patients' family and not during the informed consent procedure.

We can conclude that the Czech Republic is still behind in its development, and that it is only a matter of time until the Czech public will appreciate the informed consent institute adequately. Another possibility is to ask some questions. Informed consent has its origin in conflicts between physicians and patients and even in lawsuits between them. (Appelbaum & Meisel, 1987) We do not remember sharp conflicts between physicians and patients in the Czech Republic, lawsuits are quite rare. In our interviews patients emphasised trust as an important part of their relationship with physicians. Due to historical reasons, the division line is not between patients and physicians, but between good and bad physicians, and between good and bad health care facilities. Information about objective outcomes of Czech hospitals (mortality rates, waiting lists, etc) is still in secret. Patients themselves must assess the quality of health care providers, so the claim for a good and sensitive expert physician survives. The conversation assessment of the quality of the physician is much more important than information given. In this way the almost forgotten question of personality traits of a good physician was revived. An important reason for Czech patients not accepting informed consent could be their wish to have physicians of high quality. Through their signatures patients simply confirm that they trust their physicians or health care facilities. (Simek et al., 2009)

In theoretical reflections of the process we can refresh an old problem from medical deontology: What does it mean to be a physician of high quality? What kind of a physician can a patient trust?

There is no doubt that a good physician must be an excellent expert in biological medicine. To become a medical expert he needs a certain level of intelligence, good memory, a strong will to study hard, and later on to work hard. A physician needs a sound reason for clinical thinking and the flexibility necessary for lifelong learning.

Moreover, physicians (and nurses) constitute distinct professional communities. Some guiding principles of these communities are different from principles common in the majority of society. An important principle in health care is beneficence. It means "act in the best interest of your patient". It clearly differs from the common rule of market (and consumers) society "following your own interests will help the well-being of the whole society". A good member of the medical community should possess special skills and strengths. To this we can apply McIntyre's definition of virtues (McIntyre, 1985) in close connection with practices of the given profession or community. Explanation represents a special problem in medicine. We can revive the term of "hermeneutic competence" promoted by Dirk Lanzerath. (Lanzerath, 2003) Eventually Chris Gastmans et al. In their effort to grasp the fundamentals of nursing ethics, came to the conclusion that caring behaviour is the integration of virtue and expert activity. (Gastmans et al., 1998)

3. Issue of resource allocation, priorities in medicine, and rationing in the CR, before and after the change

Health belongs to basic needs. Health is an essential condition for fulfilling other needs and only a healthy person can follow his own personal goals. Therefore, in our Euro-Atlantic civilisation justice and equity are highly recognized values in health care. Realisation of these values is more and more difficult. Thanks to scientific and technological progress possibilities in health care grow faster than available resources. Another problem stems from big differences in economic power of various countries. Exhibiting patients' autonomy and justice in health care presuppose minimal economic standards and democratic conditions. According to the OECD report in Germany, yearly expenditures per capita are more than two times higher than in the Czech Republic (In 2008 Germany 3208 Euro, Czech republic 1528). In Romania only 687 Euro. (Lafortune, 2010) Interpretation and realisation of concepts of justice and equity must be different in different economic conditions. In less developed countries the range of health services must be smaller; its availability in big cities and in rural areas can hardly be the same. Nevertheless, not even rich countries can provide existing diagnostic and therapeutic procedures to all without any delay, and even rich countries have rationing and priority settings.

Rationing mainly describes the process of distributing scarce health care services within a population with the effect that is not sustainable to provide each patient with all health care services he/she might benefit from. From this point of view, it reflects on a universal problem of each modern health care system that is caused by a growing discrepancy between the population's health needs and disposable financial resources. Especially high-cost health care services that are conditioned by expensive technological equipment may be subject to rationing. Nowadays' "rationing is indeed international and not just a by-product of state-commanded health care systems". (Klein, 1998) Under every constitutional "right to health care", a pragmatic necessity of how to implement it is hidden. Due to limited resources, rationing requires the selection of the best indicated patients, or putting the patients on a waiting list. The economic situation of the particular country only makes this strain either smaller or greater.

It is necessary to distinguish between political and economic decisions on macro- and/or mesolevel and professional medical assessment of health needs and clinical decision-making in the course of therapy at the microlevel (Michaeli, 1999), while both are interfering with each other. For politicians it is not popular to inform the public about urgent limitation of care for financial reasons, because of fear of social tensions and public protests that usually follow such political statements. Confrontation of these two perspectives - the political/economical one with that of medicine - leads to a conflict of interests that can be reduced by specific agreements between politicians and physicians.

With regard to the rules, two forms of rationing may be distinguished. Explicit rationing relies on clearly defined indicators and rules, while implicit rationing is based on non-obvious intra-professional norms and rules that are elaborated by medical professionals themselves. Explicit rationing presupposes an open information exchange and usually leads to the dissatisfaction of the population. Apart from the negative social impact, the tendency of explicit rules leading to a strict standardisation in health care provision and low sensitiveness to individual patient's differences may be another disadvantage. D. Mechanic says that "explicit guidelines are likely to fall short relative to the complexity of circumstances surrounding serious illness, or to be so detailed that they are impracticable" (Mechanic, 1995). Explicit rules promise distinctive transparency and accountability in medical decision-making, nevertheless, there is no doubt that aggressive interventions of economists or managers in a regulatory way may be counterproductive.

Implicit rationing usually results from a controlled supply and limited technological equipment, and is traditionally managed by means of waiting lists or denial of care. The professional assessment of health needs and medical prognosis often includes judgement of intelligence, family circumstances (hygiene), social status, profession, and/or personality traits. Physicians are supposed to be the best-qualified persons to decide for the provision of health care services. The fundamental value that is rooted in the background of implicit rationing is the deepest trust between the physician and his patients. Disadvantage of implicit rationing is its discreteness and loss of public control over the medical decisions. It can lead to a false social illusion about universal rights to health. In vulnerable societies (like the transition societies in Central and Eastern Europe), the black market can govern the distribution mechanisms. Assertive patients (better educated, rich, powerful, and motivated) may be preferred. Social bias naturally contradicts the traditional ethical principles of medical profession; that is why physicians do not like admitting that social factors intervene in their decision-making process. Therefore, in spite of the fact that the selection process includes social bias, decisions only use medical argumentation.

In practice, rationing requires a mix of explicit and implicit rules. Despite the fact that explicit rationing has recently been advocated as more appropriate (equitable and efficient), implicit rules of rationing can be, in fact, more equitable than formal explicit rules, because they can respect concrete individual circumstances (e.g. disparity between chronological and biological age). On the other hand,"making the clinician responsible for rationing puts too much power in one person's hand" (Ellis, 1999). Knowing the double responsibility of each physician - to patients as individuals and to the community as a whole - makes the patients unsure about the advice they are receiving. And finally, a feeling of justice in democratic society is principally connected with equal chances, transparency, accountability, and public control. As Robert Spaemann (Spaemann, 1995) says,"Being dependent in the matter of justice on the fact, that the other will be fair is contradictory to the fundamental requirement of symmetry."

Czech people experienced two opposite systems of financing health care. First, a seriously underfinanced and paternalistic communist state system hiding all troubles connected with lack of resources. Political propaganda promised free health care for everybody and high scientific quality. In everyday experiences people very soon realised that all these promises are impossible to fulfil. In the eighties a joke circulated rewording a classical fairytale. The joke well illustrates the experiences of Czech people with state health care regardless of state propaganda. "Socialist health care was born and a big christening party was held. Three strange sisters were invited, the fourth was forgotten. The first strange sister declared "you will be free" the second "you will be for everybody" and the third declared "you will be of highest scientific quality". Then the forgotten strange sister arrived. She could not change the previous prophecies, so she declared: "it never will be that all three prophecies will be in force simultaneously. At least one will always be missing." The Czech experiences correspond with this joke. Health care, which was free for everybody, was not of the highest quality; new expensive technology was not for everybody and many patients were obliged to pay for it. Grey economy became a stable part of health care.

People's attitudes differed. Many citizens expressed dissatisfaction with the grey economy and with difficult accession to modern health services. But there were many patients who did not bribe physicians and did not show any dissatisfaction. Some of them believed that the Czech health care is excellent, because they did not see any other possibility. Some people considered health care to be a component of human fate. When one was in the right time at the right place, he/she was lucky and could survive. If not, it was a matter of bad luck as many other fatal situations. In paternalistic society physicians were powerful agents and the best way how to get their favour was a bribe. The bribe could be financial or in the form of some scarce service. Some goods and services were hardly available. People who could offer something to mutual exchange had a much better life than others. Physicians belonged to this privileged group and so their social status was quite high. In spite of this, the majority of physicians was not satisfied. The permanent search for scarce technology was exhausting, and the grey economy was obviously in conflict with Hippocratic tradition. It is no wonder that the decision of the Czech government to move to insurance system was almost consensually accepted.

In 1992 a public health insurance system was introduced. Very soon it appeared that the modern health care system is rooted in democratic negotiations. Many problems began to be addressed publicly and public negotiation about possibilities to solve indentified problems began. All beliefs in other possibility to solve problems gradually appeared to be false. Initially, Czech political leaders believed in market forces and state interventions were not popular. The insurance system has many market elements; therefore, the Czech political leaders believed that the system will work well without any regulatory interventions. Only a strike of physicians in 1994 forced the Czech politicians to take the risk of breaking down the Czech health care seriously. (Šimek, 1996) Negotiations between health care providers, insurance companies, and state officials began, and have lasted until now under the heading of "tripartite."

In the early phases after the introduction of the insurance system in financing health care in the Czech Republic, Czech physicians exhibited quite high moral standards. As we mentioned earlier, in the first several years after the implementation of the system in Czech health care, an enormous amount of money was spent in the system without any efficient control. Czech physicians did not misuse relative free available resources for private profits. New modern technology and scarce drugs were purchased without notable regard on the physician's incomes. The physicians' strike in 1994 was not so much a demand for a raise of wages; much more important stimulus was the need to rationalise the flow of money in health care. In that time "salus aegroti" was really the "suprema lex".

An increasing gap between the financial resources (collected by public health insurance) and skyrocketing health care costs have required some urgent regulatory measures. Finally, some restrictions in the supply of health services were implemented. In 1997, ambulatory specialists were given an upper limit of incomes and general practitioners shifted to capitation fee (complemented by fees for special services). In hospitals, fixed budgets have been re-established according to the sum and structure of health care services provided in the previous period (called"historic limits from 1996-1997"). (Krizova & Simek, 2002)

While the first transformation period was accompanied with the boom of Western hi-tech medical care, the shift to prospective payments with upper limits has frozen the escalation of volume of care, and even led to a decrease in provided services in some hospitals. According to data provided by The General Health Insurance Company (GHIC), the volume of hospital services fell immediately to 80% on average while the minimum rate being set by the payer (GHIC) was 75% of the entire volume. Physicians warned the public that it would be no longer possible to achieve the same quality and accessibility of care. Rationing has become a matter of broad mass media campaign. Hospital departments, hospitals, or individual physicians have tried to compensate for their losses by "non-profit charity foundations". Patients, citizens, or corporate donors can subsidise the clinical care by contributions to these charities. It is not unlikely that this sponsoring had influenced access to services that were restricted by waiting time or denial - especially hip replacement, cardio surgery, eye treatment etc. Some physicians admitted that they had somehow taken the fact of sponsoring into account in course of their clinical decision-making. Nevertheless, in their opinion, "they always try to balance the health needs of different patients and not to harm patients in acute need". According to the official statement of the Czech Medical Chamber, sponsoring must not have any influence on the provision of health care services and must not be negotiated at the moment of acute health need.

A special form of sponsoring was organised by private providers who had asked their patients to pay an extra annual registration fee. They pointed out higher investments to their medical practice and better equipment. The fact that some patients do pay these fees may have an impact on medical decisions about referrals to specialists, spa treatment, rehabilitation, psychotherapy or prescription of expensive drugs. The patients may be differentiated by the fact that they showed their loyalty to their physician by registration fees. The way the doctor assesses their medical need becomes influenced by financial incentives and it is not excluded, that the economic motivation of the physician may slightly change his/her clinical view.

Concerning the most expensive technology and treatment, several therapies (e.g. cochlear and pacemaker implants, neuromodulation treatment in epileptic patients, betapherone treatment in sclerosis multiplex) have recently been regulated by a special commission. This care is financed separately from the budgetary scheme. The payment is sent directly from a special fund of the health insurance company to the hospital. The commission is competent to review the professional indication and upon its acceptance it issues a final approval of the health care provision. The commissioners come from health insurance funds, clinical facilities, the Health Ministry, and the public. The major power is given to the professional medical assessment of the patients' health condition. Only those patients who have already been selected in previous steps by medical professionals are submitted for the more or less formal approval by the commission. Social characteristics may play a certain role; nevertheless, no patient is a priority discriminated on grounds of their social or ethnic origin.

From the beginning of 2008 after the amendment of Act No. 48/1997 Sb., "on the public health insurance" some patients' copayments were introduced. It was a small regulatory fee (30 Czech crowns, a little more than 1 Euro) for clinical examination and a larger fee (90 Czech crowns, almost 4 Euro) for examination at emergency units and charge for each day of hospitalisation (60 Czech crowns, 2.5 Euro). This legal provision provoked sharp political discussion with quite common lack of sound arguments on both sides. In an apparent conflict with law some social democratic county representatives even paid charges for patients in district hospitals from other sources. Nevertheless, the fees brought remarkable sum of money in health care institutes.

To sum it up, in the Czech Republic there are two ways how to overcome difficulties in covering health care expenditures. One is slow introduction of co-payments, both by political decisions and by private initiative of health care institutions. The second is rationing (or priority setting). The political part of rationing is mainly realised through setting economic limits for health care institutions. Economic limits result in two restrictions. The well visible restrictions are waiting lists which have become the standard part of medical care. The less observable restriction represents slower introduction of new technology.

A good example of gradual introduction of advanced technology in accordance with available resources is the distribution of Percutaneous Transluminal Coronary Angioplasty (PTCA) in the Czech Republic. Percutaneous Transluminal Coronary Angioplasty (PTCA) is an effective reperfusion strategy in acute myocardial infarction. Its introduction in therapeutic practice was an important achievement, which helped to dramatically decrease in-hospital mortality from acute myocardial infarction in the last two decades of the twentieth century. In the Czech Republic the first PTCA was done in 1981. In 1999 the method was available only in big prominent centres and for many patients it was not available. Then the four angioplasty centres (they routinely used primary coronary angioplasty from 1995) asked the question how to offer the life saving method also to patients from areas where there were no angioplasty centres. The Cardiocenter of University Hospital Vinohrady, Prague, coordinated a well known and frequently cited study assessing the safety of transporting patients to an angioplasty centre. Transferring patients from community hospitals to a tertiary angioplasty centre in the acute phase of myocardial infarction was proved to be feasible and safe. (Widimský et al., 2000)

In 2000 we did research on the equity in availability of PTCA. It was just proved that transport is safe and life saving, so we asked on distribution of performed PTCAs in the Czech Republic and on practices of transports to angioplasty centres. (Not yet published data.)

There were dramatic differences in performed PTCAs between regions in the Czech Republic. In Prague patients there were performed 3 678 PTCAs, it is 58.4% of all PTCAs performed. It means 306 PTCAs done on 100 000 inhabitants. In patients from Southern Bohemia only 173 PTCAs were done, it is 2.7% of all PTCAs and 24.7 PTCAs done on 100 000 inhabitants.

In the second step we made a simple questionnaire survey among Czech physicians. (Final sample was 401 physicians, response rate was 26.7%.) We asked them about the availability of PTCA, about the reasons why some patients do not receive PTCA treatment, and finally, how important informal relationships between physicians in charge are.

The majority of responding physicians (71.4% yes and probably yes) considered PTCA available, only 28.6% of physicians answered no and probably no. There were significant differences between physicians from big cities and from other sites. 89.2% of those who answered no and probably no on the question on availability were physicians from other sites.

We offered several reasons why some of their patients did not receive PTCA treatment. Respondents from big cities preferred the response "the patient came to the specialised centre late" while respondents from other sites preferred response "the patient was referred to a hospital where PTCA is not performed".

As to the impact of informal relationships between physicians on referral to specialised centre 14.2% of respondents consider it very strong, 32.8% respondents somehow strong, 30% of respondents think that informal relationships are probably not important and only 10.1% of respondents are sure that informal relationships have no impact on referral of patients with myocardial infarction.

Results of our research illustrate the process of development of new expensive technology in dependence on available resources. In the first stage new technology is available only at the big centres and there could not be equity in its distribution. In this stage physicians are aware of the lack of equity, and they are searching for ways to do the process more equitably. Chance and informal relationships of the patient and his attending physician often play an important role in the availability of the therapeutic procedure. The length of the first stage depends on the economic condition of the country, and on the pressure from experts and from members of civic society (patients' initiatives, media, etc.). There is a difficult ethical dilemma in the situation. Should physicians actively announce to individual patients and the media that there is a lack of expensive life-saving technology? On one hand it is necessary to move things ahead; on the other hand, many people would get information about treatment that they never could use. In any case, at least the experts and politicians should be aware of existing life saving expensive technology on the basis of serious methods of technology assessment. Explicit health care policy should be developed and priorities openly discussed. According to our experiences here are the weak points of development in post-communist countries.

4. Institutions of ethics – The case of ethics committees

Due to historical reasons the authority of Churches is traditionally weak in the Czech society, and the Czech Republic belongs to one of the most atheistic countries in EU.

According to the Eurobarometer from June 2005 only 19% of Czech citizens agree with the statement "I believe there is a God". In the EU this percentage is only smaller in Estonia (16%) than in the Czech Republic. 30% of Czech citizens agree that „I don' t believe there is any sort of spirit, God or life force". In EU only in France more citizens (33%) agree with that statement. (Eurobarometer, 2005) In the Czech history Catholic Church was the pillar of unwanted Habsburg monarchy, Protestantism was the religion of traditional national rivals of Czech people, and so the national Renaissance in the 19th century was based on secular education and science. This tendency was to strengthen by a communist regime. Moreover, communist ideology based on Marxist philosophy did not elaborate ethics as a special discipline. For these two reasons ethics as a discipline is undervalued in the Czech Republic. Common Czech people have no ethical language to use in everyday communication, and moral arguments are used rarely.

We could be worried about human relations in a society where there are no recognized experts in ethics, and people do not use the language of ethics. Our experiences are not fatal, ethical behaviour survives even under such conditions. On the contrary, in an ascribed situation natural moral processes are more visible. We can watch the emergence of moral rules in natural groups and the free choice as the key element in acceptance of moral attitudes in Tugendhat sense. (Tugendhat, 1993) We experience an important role of the nuclear family in moral development. Discursive nature of contemporary ethics is also well observable, as well as troubles arising from breakdowns of the discursive process. Common people usually live in their own moral space and if asked, they most often reason their moral behaviour in terms of the golden rule. ("One should not treat others in a way that he would not like to be treated.") By using the golden rule they are also able to exhibit basic levels of abstraction.

As a result of the situation, political and scientific interest in ethics is also very low. For example there are no chairs for ethics at Czech schools of philosophy and people from religious groups in a new generation of health care ethics teachers prevail. Paradoxically, in the most atheistic country of the EU, in majority of (a few) leading positions in health care ethics are theologists and catholic priests. So the only really secular institutions which are explicitly working in the area of ethics are ethics committees. Ethics committees constitute a special new version of ethical community. They represent a rare social group in the Czech Republic, where the language of ethics is used, and ethics is the matter of concern. Members of ethics committees intuitively use basic tools of contemporary ethics - plurality of attitudes, discourse, and search for consensus. For this reason ethics committees attracted our attention and we did some research on their functioning in the Czech Republic. (Šimek et al., 2008)

The ethics committees are currently remarkable institutions. They function as an authority - without their approval it is not possible to do any clinical research study. On the contrary to common authorities they do not arrive at their decisions on the basis of application of definite general rules, but through methods of ethical discourse. (Whittaker, 2005) They are relatively new institutions; the first recommendation to establish ethics committees at research institutes comes from the first revision of the Declaration of Helsinki in 1975. Therefore, there are many uncertainties in understanding their role and function and we can find some studies concerning a comparison of formal aspects of work of the ethics committees in various states of the EU (Davies et al., 2009; EFGCP Ethics Working Party,

2007; Hedgecoe et al., 2006), historical works (Glasa, 2000; Hedgecoe, 2009) or detailed analyses of some of the (discursive) practices of the ethics committees (Angell et al., 2006; O´Reilly et al., 2009).

In the Czech Republic the ethics committees were only created in 1990. It was the initiative of Martin Bojar, then the Minister of Health. He established the Central Ethics Committee at the Ministry of Health, and recommended to all major health institutions to create their local ethics committees. Within a short period of time 20 local ethics committees were established and their number has gradually grown to the current number of approximately 100. (Simek, 2000) Functions were voluntary and unpaid, and the main qualification was the moral credit of appointed volunteers. Until the adoption of Act No. 79/1997 Coll. on medicines, the Czech ethics committees had been operating without any statutory regulation for many years. (Šimek et al., 2000) In the year 2004 the Directive 2001/20/EC was incorporated into the Czech legislation (current legislation: Act No. 378/2007 Coll. on medicines and Decree No. 226/2008 Coll.). In 2003, under the new legislation, some local ethics committees were recognized by the Ministry of Health as multi-centric ethics committees. Their task is to provide a single national opinion on multi-centric clinical studies. The local ethics committees continue to express their views on mono-centric studies, and give their opinion on the appropriateness of carrying out an authorized multi-centric study in the place under their authority. (Šimek et al., 2008)

Our research started by participatory observation at meetings and at the Summer Schools of Medical Ethics, organized by the Forum of Czech Ethics Committees. Furthermore, we carried out half-structured interviews with the members of the ethics committees, with representatives of contracting authorities, with examining doctors (investigators), and 1 interview with a representative of the State Office for Drug Control. Six focus groups were organized with the members of the ethics committees. To get an overview of the distribution of some of the attitudes expressed in the interviews, a simple questionnaire survey was realized among the members of the ethics committees. The response rate was 11 % so it was only of an illustrative nature.

If we try to generalize our experience, the members of the Czech ethics committees are people willing to selflessly do something more for the "common good". They are not authoritarian in their role; they prefer agreement over all other possibilities of conflict resolution. Like in other European countries (Klingmann, 2009) only about 1% of studies is rejected. Significantly, more frequent are comments intended to modify a project, about one half of projects are adjusted based on comments from an ethics committee. In the interviews and discussions the members agreed that they feel better in the role of an advisor rather than an arbiter.

The chairman of the committee usually has natural authority. The next important person is the secretary. S/he is the guarantee of an error-free bureaucratic part of the work. Discussions of the committee are sometimes more, sometimes less discursive and usually take place in an atmosphere of tolerance; anyone who so desires is given an opportunity to express his/her opinion on the discussed matter. Most often the resolution is adopted by consensus, only rarely is it necessary to vote. Remuneration for the work was never raised as an important issue.

Most members of the ethics committees are health professionals. Laymen (most often theologists, lawyers, civil servants) are members of a committee mainly because the law requires it. The relationship of the health professionals towards the laymen is friendly, but it is possible to see some reluctance of the ethics committees to accept a larger number of lay members. This is not unusual for the Czech Republic. A similar situation was noted in a Dutch study (Caron-Flinterman et al., 2009) and it is possible to notice a call for greater involvement of patients and their organizations that are already in the preparation of clinical trials. (Wrobel, 2009)

There are certainly many reasons for this hesitation. The common basis we see in uncertainties and tensions faced by the ethics committees. (Barke, 2009) A good clinical trial proves common laws valid for everybody, a good care wants to improve the health and quality of life of an individual patient. (Mol, 2006) The ECs members might feel that there is too much that they are not able to control when they assess the ethical legitimacy of a clinical trial application. (DeMets et al., 2006; Tailor et al. 2008) Given the absence of pre-given answers, the ECs have to actively construct what counts as (an) ethical (issue). The legitimacy of their arguments and decisions is built on heterogeneous sources and performs various functions. (O´Reilly et al., 2009)

The health professionals usually see the benefit of the ill in maintaining or improving their biological health. It is true that preservation of biological life and health is the most crucial task of contemporary health care systems, but the benefit of the ill can be viewed from many different perspectives. (Mol, 2002) We can understand that the health professionals' hesitation to accept the laymen among themselves could also be caused by their fear that other views on the benefit of the ill could prevail in the discussion.

Another common characteristic of the members of the ethics committees is their problem to explain in detail, why they do their work, and what it brings them. When asked questions on their motivation for being members of an EC, respondents felt uncertain and uneasy. Answers were usually very poor and largely formal. The members of the ethics committees most frequently named the necessity and usefulness of their work, without specifying in what exactly they see this necessity and usefulness. Education is not recognized as an important aid. In the interviews the need for education was never mentioned spontaneously. Maybe the controversial role of the ethics committees is reflected here. It is very difficult to be an ethical body and an office at the same time. Underscoring the importance of education shows that members of the Czech ECs do not get the message from the outside world that the controversy of their role can be resolved through education.

In 2005 the civil association, the Forum of Czech Ethics Committees, was established. Twice a year the Forum organizes discussion meetings, and in the summer, the School of Medical Ethics. About fifty people take part in these activities. Participation in the discussion meetings is not formal; the members of the ethics committees come with a visible interest in the matter, and they vividly discuss topics of their interest. Even at these discussions there is an atmosphere of an unusual tolerance. Although opinions sometimes largely differ, serious disputes do not arise.

From a theoretical perspective we can see the Czech ethics committees as more or less informal communities of people having similar sets of attitudes, tasks, and practicalities.

Contemporary sociology offers some concepts that could help us better understand what is going on (or could be) in the development of ethics committees. (Simek et al., 2010)

Ethics committees could be understood as an ethical community. An ethical community is originally the concept of I. Kant. (Kant, 1996) (Wood, 2000) We cannot fully apply the whole concept; instead, it could be an inspiration for us. The term could be used only in a weak sense.

In the current world of secularization and globalization, religious communities lose their strong influence. People who share the same values rather create informal groups or communities. The members of the ethics committees form a community of people willing to devote a bit of their time and effort to the common good. Their participation comes from free decision, and their motivation is largely moral. In their effort they do not seek prestige or material benefit. In this sense, the members of the ethics committees fulfil some of the characteristics of Kant's "ethical community". There are also substantial differences. Kantian ethics is based on duty, to be a member of an ethics committee is a free choice. Religious position is not the unifying element. A community of ethics committees' members is not and will not be universalistic; it will be bound to a particular common task and to a particular common area. The unifying element of this community is a common specific work task - the protection of subjects of clinical trials.

Another concept that could be applied is the concept of epistemic community. Peter M. Haas defines an epistemic community as "a network of professionals with recognized expertise in a particular domain and an authoritative claim to policy-relevant knowledge within that domain". (Haas, 1992) There are four elements in his definition and the Czech ethics committees fulfil two of them.

They have a shared set of normative and principled beliefs which provide a value-base rationale for the social actions of community members (principles of the Good Clinical Practice and related codes and legislation). In the ethics committees one can observe a common policy enterprise - that is, a common set of practices associated with a set of problems to which their professional competence is directed, presumably out of the conviction that as a result, human welfare will be enhanced.

The other two points of the definition - shared causal beliefs and shared notions of validity - are fulfilled by scientists and experts in the ethics, who, on an all-European scale, work together to define principles of the current research ethics. These experts meet and discuss at preparation of documents, as well as at various conferences, and they publish in professional journals. In this way they create an epistemic basis for addressing the problems of security and preservation of human dignity of the research subjects. (Salter & Jones, 2005)

The Czech ethics committees can be considered a local embodiment of the international epistemic community of investigators and bioethicists, who on the supranational level of European directives and international harmonization efforts defined the framework and rules of their operation.

The last inspiration we can find in the concept of communities of practice. (Wenger & Snyder, 2000) The communities of practice are characterized by three main features: 1) interest and even passion for a particular area, 2) community - they engage in joint meetings and discussions, help each other, and share information, build mutual relationships, meet both in person and "online", and 3) experience and practices - they are united not only by the interest in the same thing, but also by sharing sets of conduct, by the way they deal with things and situations, by the effort to learn to do things differently, to learn things they care about, to do better.

The ethics committees basically operate on these principles. Within the framework of the regular meetings organized by the Forum of Ethics Committees as well as email conferences and website administering, there is an exchange of views, a mutual enrichment, and learning from the experience of others. Discussions are often vivid, and the ethics committees do not agree on many things. However, they share the effort to change something, to learn from each other, and to improve. They also enter into discussions with those from the "other side", with the contracting authorities, and these discussions are interesting and beneficial for both parties.

The ethics committees are new institutions and their roles and functioning are not yet fully stabilized. The basic existential dilemma is their dual role. It is not easy to keep balance between the role of the ethical agents and the role of officials and experts. Moreover, the role of an ethical agent is difficult. Ethics committees assist at keeping ethical standards in the field of continually developing clinical research. For this they need a certain range of knowledge, but also ethical creativity. By ethical creativity we mean an ability to apply, in a creative way, recognized principles of good clinical practice in new unexpected situations. It must be rooted in ethical honesty; creativity can have different meanings.

The ethics committees are, and will increasingly be, under pressure for transparency and accountability of their work, and they will have to open to a greater number of laymen. (Avard et al., 2009; Kelly, 2003) This represents a challenge for the future. The members of ethics committees will need to better elaborate the discursive part of their work. They should better understand what they are doing and why they do it. They should learn to use arguments to justify their standpoints and decisions.

Here are reasons why they will need a good education even if they underscore it. We attempted to apply the concepts of the epistemic community, the ethical community, and the community of practice to the phenomenon of ethics committees. It offers certain concepts, perhaps visions, which could become a functional basis for a discussion about the role of the ethics committees in the near future.

5. Conclusions

Medical ethics is a Cinderella among other medical disciplines, but in a synergy with other forces (EU legislation, international contacts, development of components of civic society) it has some impact on the development in the Czech Republic. As a discipline, medical ethics suffers from lack of experts, insufficient amount of research projects, public presentation, periodicals, and publications. Medical ethicists are not considered to be relevant stakeholders in health policy making or in discussions on the shape of the Czech health care system. Positively, it has been established at each medical faculty and now it is an obligatory part of health care providers' education. Some research was done and interested persons meet at conferences and seminars. In our survey we presented some results of ten years' research.

Informed consent was in the Czech Republic implemented from above (EU legislation) and without previous discussions among stakeholders. For this reason it is often understood as a mere formal instrument. Due to historical reasons everyday democratic negotiation is not well developed, and therefore, shared decision making is not an issue in discussions about the implementations of informed consent in the Czech health care. In this specific context the call for a reliable and trustworthy physician is better visible.

Rationing in the Czech Republic has its specific features thanks to a more prominent lack of resources and thanks to the transition from a paternalistic state health care system to democratic insurance based system. It took some time to understand the need for implementation of regulative measures in the system. Only gradually did all the stakeholders learn the need for negotiations. Official co-payments of patients were unusual and their acceptance in public was quite difficult. Public debate was too much emotive and lacked sound arguments. We could also notice how the slowing down of high expensive technology development could help to overcome deficiencies in resources.

Ethics committees in the Czech Republic represent a special institute of secular ethics in the country, where ethics is underscored both in academia and in everyday communication. We propose to use concepts of ethical community, epistemic community, and community of practice, to better understand the role and mission of ethics committees.

Funding: The research project is supported by the Grant Agency of the Czech Republic (GA CR), contract No. P407/11/0380

6. References

Angell E., Sutton AJ., Windridge K., Dison-Woods M. (2006) Consistency in decision making by research ethics committees: a controlled comparison *J Med Ethics* 2006;32: pp. 662-664

Appelbaum PS., Meisel A. (1987): *Informed consent: legal theory and clinical practice.* New York: Oxford Univ. Press.

Avard D., Stanton-Jean M., Woodgate R.L., Pullman D., Sagimur R. (2009). Research Ethics Boards and challenges for public participation. *Health Law Rev ;17,2-3* , pp. 66-73.

Barke, R. (2009). Balancing uncertain risks and benefits in human subjects research. *Sci Technol Human Values;34* , pp. 337-364.

Caron-Flinterman JL, Broerse JEW, Bunders JFG. (2009): Patient partnership in decision-making on biomedical research: Changing the network. *Sci Technol Human Values*;32: pp. 339-368.

Davies H, Wells F, Czarkowski M (2009): Standards for research ethics committees: purpose, problems and the possibilities of other approaches. *J Med Ethics; 35,6,* pp. 382-383.

DeMets D L, Fost N, Powers M. (2006): An Institutional Review Board dilemma: Responsible for safety monitoring but not in control. *Clin Trials* 2006;3: pp.142-148

EFGCP (Europen Forum for good Clinical Practice) Ethics Working Party. (2007): The procedure for the ethical review of protocols for clinical research projects in the European Union. *Int J Pharm Med; 21,1* , pp. 3-113.

Ellis, S. (1999). Fidelity and stewardship are incompatible when attempted by same individual. *British Medical Journal 318 (7188)* , p. 940.

Eurobarometer June 2005: *Social values, Science and Technology.*

Gastmans Ch., Schotmans P., Deirckx de Casterle B. (1998). Nursing considered as Moral Practice. A philosophical-ethical interpretation of Nursing. *Kennedy Institute of Ethics Journal, 8* , pp. 43-69.

Glasa, J. (. (2000). *Ethics Committees in Central & Eastern Europe - Present State & Perspectives for the 21st Century". Conference proceedings.* Bratislava.

Haas, P. (1992). Introduction: epistemic communities and international policy coordination. :. *Int Organ;46,1* , pp. 1-35.

Hedgecoe A., Carvalho F., Lobmayer P., Raka F. (2006). Research ethics committees in Europe: implementing the directive, respecting diversity. *J Med Ethics;32*, pp. 483-486.

Hedgecoe, A. (2009). "A Form of Practical Machinery": The Origins of Research Ethics Committees in the UK, 1967–1972. *Med Hist;53, 3*, pp. 331–350.

Haškovcová, H. (2002). *Lékařská etika. (Medical Ethics).* Praha : Galén

Kant, I. (1996). *Religion within the Boundaries of Mere Reason (Religion inerhalb des bloßen Vernunft).* Cambridge: Cambridge University Press

Kelly, S. (2003). Public Bioethics and publics: Consensus, boundaries and Participation in Biomedical science policy. *Sci Technol Human Values ;28*, pp. 339-364.

Klein, R. (1998). Puzzling out priorities. *British Medical Journal 317 (7188)* , pp. 959

Klingmann I. (Project Coordinator) Impact on Clinical Research of European Legislation. HEALTH-F1-2007-201002, Project Final Report. EFGCP, February 2009. http://www.efgcp.be/downloads/icrel_docs/Final_report_ICREL.pdf (accessed January 2012)

Krizova, E., Simek, J.(2002): Rationing of expensive medical care in a transition country - nihil novum? *J.Med.Ethics*, 28, pp. 308-312

Krizova, E., Simek, J. (2007): Theory and practice of informed consent in the Czech Republic *J Med Ethics*, 33: pp. 273-277.

Lafortune, G. d. (2010). *Health at a Glance: Europe 2010.* OECD.

Lanzerath, D. (2003). Ethics in Genetics: The Use of Genetic Knowledge – Remarks on the hermeneutic competence in genetic counselling. *International Conference on Bioethics in Central and Eastern Europe 11-12 November 2002, Vilnius, Lithuania.*

McIntyre, A. (1985). *After Virtue. A Study in Moral Theory.* London: Duckworth

Mechanic, D. (1995). Dilemmas in rationing health care services: the case for implicit rationing. *British Medical Journal 310* , pp. 1655 - 1659.

Michaeli, D. (1999). Rationing is a two-level process. *British Medical Journal 318 (7188)*, p. 940.

Mol, A. (2002). *Body multiple: Ontology in Medical practice.* Durham: Duke University Press.

Mol A. (2006): Proving or improving: On health care research as a form of self-reflection. *Qual Health Res;* 16: pp.405-414

O'Reilly M., Dixon-Woods M., Angell E., Ashcroft R., Bryman A. (2009). Doing accountability: a discourse analysis of research ethics committee letters. *Sociol Health Iln;31,2*, pp. 246-261.

Salter B, Jones M. (2005): Biobanks and bioethics: The politics of legitimation. *Journal of European Public Policy ;12,4* , pp. 710-732.

Simek, J. (1999): The Right to Health Care in the Post-Totalitarien Czech Republic. In D. a. Exter, *The Right to Health Care in Several European Countries.* London: Kluwer Law International.

Simek, J. (2000). History and Function of Newly Established Ethics Committees in the Czech Republic. V H. Hofmeister, *Der Mensch als Subjekt und Objekt der Medizin.* Neukirchener ver.

Šimek J, Šilhanová J, Vrbatová I. (2000): Ethics Committees in Czech Republic. In Glasa J., ed. *Ethics Committees in Central & Eastern Europe - Present State & Perspectives for the 21st Century.* Conference proceedings. Bratislava.

Šimek L, Zamykalová L., Mesanyová M. Etické komise v České republice. (Ethics committees in the Czech Republic) *Prakt. Lék.* 2008, 88, No. 1, pp. 3-5

Simek, J., Krizová, E., Zamykalová, L. Mesanyová, M. (2009): *Informed Consent, Trust and Virtue in Czech Medicine* Ethics, Law and Society. Vol. IV., Ashgate, London. March 2009 pp. 237 - 246

Simek, J., Zamykalova, L., Mesanyova, M. (2010): Ethics Committee or Community? Examining the Identity of Czech Ethics Committees in the Period of Transition. *J.Med.Ethics,* 36 (9), pp. 548-552

Spaemann, R. (1995). *Základní mravní pojmy. ("Elementary concepts of ethics").* Praha: Svoboda.

Tailor HA, Chaisson L, Sugarman J. (2008): Enhancing communication among data monitoring committee and institutional review boards. *Clin Trials;*5: pp.277-282

Tugendhat, E. (1993). *Vorlesungen über Ethik.* Frankfurt am Main: Suhrkamp.

Whittaker, E. (2005). Adjudicating entitlements: The emerging discourses of research ethics boards. *Healt ;9* , pp. 513-535.

Widimský P, Groch L, Zelízko M, Aschermann M, Bednár F, Suryapranata H. (2000): Multicentre randomized trial comparing transport to primary angioplasty vs immediate thrombolysis vs combined strategy for patients with acute myocardial infarction presenting to a community hospital without a catheterization laboratory. The PRAGUE study. *Eur Heart J.* May; 21(10): pp.823-31.

Wenger E, Snyder W. (2000). Communities of practice: The organizational frontier. *Harv Bus Rev,* (January-February) pp. 139-145.

Wood, A. (2000). Religion, Ethical Community and the Struggle against Evil. *Faith Philos;17,* pp. 498-511.

Wrobel, E. (2009). *Report. EPPOSI Workshop On Clinical Trials. Shaping the future of European Clinical Trial Legislation.* Brussels: EPPOSI (European Platform for Patient's Organisations, Science and Industry)

Zamykalová, L., Šimek, J. (2007): Informovaný souhlas v praxi na českých klinikách. (Informed consent in practice at the Czech clinics) *Prakt. Lék.*, 87, No. 7, pp. 406-413